DATE DUE

Praise for
Who's Afraid of Human Cloning?
by Gregory E. Pence

"Thoughtfully written and persuasive . . . recommended for all readers."
—*Choice*

"The best thing written about cloning since the birth of Dolly. . . .A penetrating analysis."
—*Skeptical Inquirer*

"An important, largely rational, and informative account."
—*San Francisco Chronicle*

"A rattling good polemic against the rush to condemn human cloning."
—*New Scientist*

"This book evokes a sigh of relief."
—*Booklist*

"The antidote to the hysterical, irrational, and just plain false information about human cloning from the popular press."
—*RESOLVE Newsletter*
(for infertile couples)

RE-CREATING MEDICINE

RE-CREATING MEDICINE

Ethical Issues at the
Frontiers of Medicine

Gregory E. Pence

ROWMAN & LITTLEFIELD PUBLISHERS, INC.
Lanham • Boulder • New York • Oxford

ROWMAN & LITTLEFIELD PUBLISHERS, INC.

Published in the United States of America
by Rowman & Littlefield Publishers, Inc.
4720 Boston Way, Lanham, Maryland 20706
http://www.rowmanlittlefield.com

12 Hid's Copse Road
Cumnor Hill, Oxford OX2 9JJ, England

British Library Cataloguing in Publication Information Available

Library of Congress Cataloging-in-Publication Data

Pence, Gregory E.
  Re-creating medicine : ethical issues at the frontiers of medicine / Gregory E. Pence.
    p. cm.
  Includes bibliographical references and index.
  ISBN 0-8476-9690-1 (alk. paper)
  1. Medical innovations—Moral and ethical aspects. I. Title.
  [DNLM: 1. Ethics, Medical. 2. Bioethics. 3. Genetic Engineering. W 50 P397r 2000]
  R725.5 .P46 2000
  174'.25—dc21

                                                        99-086178

Printed in the United States of America

⊗™ The paper used in this publication meets the minimum requirements of
American National Standard for Information Sciences—Permanence of Paper for
Printed Library Materials, ANSI/NISO Z39.48–1992.

CONTENTS

ACKNOWLEDGMENTS

There are four special people to whom I owe a particular debt in the writing of this book. Fellow UAB (University of Alabama at Birmingham) philosophy professors Ted Benditt and Mary Whall read everything I gave them and were very generous with their time and comments. Kelly Smith of Clemson University was the ideal outside reviewer, commenting on every page and greatly improving the book. The engaged minds of these three astute reviewers each made their mark on this book in big ways that they and I know: I am in their long-term debt. Finally, my B.S./M.D. research assistant for the summer of 1999, Jason Lott, was indispensable in producing this book. Together, we both learned in researching the book, and we learned from each other.

Dennis Boulware, M.D. at UAB, and Laurel Simmons, founder/moderator of the internet-based, Bone Marrow Transplantation Talk (BMT-Talk), helped me learn about cybermedicine. Philosophers Scott Arnold and Jim Rachels and Chuck Patrick of the Alabama Organ Bank read and improved the chapter about compensated organ donation (Jim also read two other chapters).

Cystic fibrosis researcher Eric Sorscher, biology professor Rob Angus, and my colleague Harold Kincaid read and improved the chapter on patenting genes.

Armand Karow of the Xytex Corporation (a tissue bank), my colleague Scott Arnold, and lawyer Mark Eibert were especially generous with their comments on buying reproductive help. Karow pointed out to me that J. Marion Sims was the first U.S. physician to try artificial insemination; Tim Pennycuff at the Reynolds Historical Library helped me find original source materials by and about Sims. Victor Chin has provided several key references in assisted reproduction.

At Rowman & Littlefield, Jon Sisk and Maureen MacGrogan were extremely supportive of this project from the very start. I appreciate their support and efforts.

I refined my views on genetic choice and cloning during talks and responding to questions at Princeton University, Transylvania University (where I gave the Kenan Lecture), the Second Conference on Mammalian Cloning (Washington, D.C.), Kent State University, LaRoche University, St. Cloud University, Monash University (Australia), the University of Akron, the University of Tennessee at Chattanooga, the University of Illinois at Chicago Medical School, the University of Northeastern Ohio Medical School, the 1998 national meeting of the American Society for Human Genetics in Denver, and the national meeting of the American Society for Tissue and Bone Collection in Tampa, Florida.

At a crucial time, my colleague in the medical school and fellow course director, pediatrician, and historian of medicine, Hughes Evans, lent me many valuable books on the history of infertility and J. Marion Sims. I am in her debt for doing so on such short notice.

PREFACE

It is my intention for this book to be on the cutting edge of the new medical ethics issues of our time. At times, I champion controversial answers. This book is not a textbook in which I neutrally discuss each side and feign impartiality. Instead, I take positions on each issue, answer opponents, and try to move the discussion forward.

At the start of a new century and a new millennium, medicine confronts many new ethical issues; I hope that this book will begin that confrontation. Perhaps the book's two most important ethical issues are the impact computers have in medicine and the possibility that parents could choose the genetic traits of their children. Writers of science fiction and medical skeptics have condemned both, but I believe that each of these issues has another side that is rarely heard.

Medicine has accomplished much during the past three decades, but what stands out is how much more it could accomplish by overcoming a backward-looking, overly cautious medical ethics. Research using human embryos and stem cells could help conquer many diseases, yet researchers are stymied by reactionary opponents. In medicine itself, opposition to providing payment for the donation of organs of brain-dead relatives has resulted in many needlessly lost lives. On the edges of medicine, similar opposition to paid reproductive assistance deprives infertile couples of wanted babies and young women of meaningful employment and financial gain.

Bioethics has functioned in much the same way for the past thirty years and has been led by a small inner circle of people who define its official issues and provide the answers given by professional ethics consultants. As such, it has grown stale and needs to be re-created. This book is a step in that direction.

In addition, the book reaches beyond our present norms to discuss topics such as when it might be right to clone humans and whether medicine should attempt to make us immortal (or force us to accept our "natural" limits). In such highly charged areas, almost any answer is controversial, and the reader should expect some controversial opinions by the author about human cloning and natural limits in medicine.

1

RE-CREATING MEDICINE BY RE-CREATING MEDICAL ETHICS

Amongst medical people, a quack is a man who does new things.
—*The Illustrated American,* circa 1855, quoted in defense of physician J. Marion Sims

It is not uncommon for anthropologists, when studying primitive cultures, to encounter taboos against behaviors that were originally prohibited for justifiable reasons but that now are clearly counterproductive. Because the banned behaviors have been forbidden for so long, no questioning of them is possible.

This book challenges taboos that no longer make sense in contemporary medicine, such as prejudices against paying for transplantable organs and reproductive help, originating humans by cloning when safe to do so, allowing parents to choose traits of children, and expanding choice in enhancement medicine. This book also discusses letting the Internet empower patients, whether genes should be patentable, and a new role for bioethics, one not so adoring of the status quo.

Ethical rules arise out of a particular time and context in human history; the same is true for the ethical rules of medicine. Periodically, such rules need to be reexamined: we should not live for the rules; the rules should live for us. When they no longer do, they should be changed.

The vast majority of physicians are conservative about changing moral rules. If you are a physician in our culture, this is the way you get perceived as wise. If you are a specialist and need referrals, you had best not be perceived as radical about bioethics. American physicians make a lot of money, and making that kind of money causes people to resist change.

So there is a vacuum for bioethics to fill in questioning ethical assumptions that operate in medicine. Although this role harkens back to Socrates, not many bioethicists have embraced it. Perhaps that is why the two leading speakers at the 1999 national meeting of bioethicists quite unintentionally chose similar titles for their talks: "Why Has Bioethics Become Boring?" and "Broadening Bioethics' Agenda."[1]

Why was there a need for such talks? One answer is that bioethicists have become too timid and respectful of the present state of medicine. Stuck in a rut of their own making, they appear on television only to complain about slippery slopes, threats of new reproductive options to the family, and to chant the mantra that "technology is changing faster than our ability to understand it." In truth, this *is* a little boring.

If we look at change in medical ethics more generally, we should remember that there is always an *ethical opportunity cost* in not going forward. Worries about slippery slopes, parents wanting only perfect babies, and our becoming Nazis were appropriate at the beginning, but this is not what constitutes *all* of bioethics.

In 1860, Alabama physician J. Marion Sims inseminated wives with their husbands' sperm in attempts to overcome infertility.[2] Producing one pregnancy this way, Sims was universally condemned for trying to produce babies "unnaturally" and for assisting women to commit "adultery." (Sims later founded the specialty of gynecology and, in New York City, the first hospital for women.)

This might be just another amusing historical anecdote of how enlightened we are now compared with "way back then," were it not for the fact that Sims's idea did not become accepted in the United States until the 1960s. Thousands of couples remained barren for a century when they might have been able to have children.

The history of medicine is especially illuminating here. There have been few great improvements advocated in medicine where the proponent has not been vilified as being unprofessional, avaricious, uncaring of his patients, and immoral. When J. Marion Sims suggested that some physicians should study and treat the special problems of women, he was ridiculed for wanting to be—using terms of great derision in his time—a *male midwife* or a *women's surgeon*.

In this case and many more in the history of medicine, moral rebuke has been a weapon of harm to humanity. Louis Pasteur and Joseph Lister were accused not only of false and dangerous views but also of *immoral* views. Today, especially in controversial areas where our deepest taboos operate—in reproductive ethics and in commercializing body parts—both medicine's and society's morality need to be reexamined.

HOW WE GO WRONG

When we try to talk about changing a moral rule in medicine or elsewhere, we are often stuck in conceptual traps that prevent progress. This book will expose and attack these "ruts." Here's a preview:

1. *Conceptualizing issues in simplistic oppositions:* A long-standing pattern in medical ethics is to see complex issues in only black-or-white, simplistic ways. The twentieth-century philosopher Ludwig Wittgenstein noted that, in ongoing philosophic debates, although the first step often escapes notice, it is absolutely crucial to how the debate is conceptualized. The issues discussed in this book usually have a classic, false first step (for example, the thinking that we can only get organs donated either through pure altruism or a crass commercial market in body parts, with no in-between solutions).

2. *Olympian standards for new options:* Especially in reproductive ethics, we demand that physicians and couples using new services be saintlike in motivation, and we want guarantees of normal babies, although we tolerate almost anything in traditional, sexual reproduction.

3. *Distrust of choices of ordinary people:* When at-risk parents seek to test themselves or their embryos for genetic disease, they are instantly accused of wanting only "perfect babies." Discussion of creating better kids too often assumes that parents are improperly motivated.

4. *Confusing distributive with evaluative questions:* Opponents say we shouldn't create drugs or genetic enhancements to make smarter kids or create smarter kids by cloning, because we can't guarantee equal access to these goods. But we don't need to know how to distribute scarce, life-saving dialysis machines to know that they are good. These are separate questions.

5. *Demonization of new inventions as "technology":* New machines (computers) or new ways of creating families are seen as threats to our humanity, rather than as expressions of it. More often, new inventions are just neutral tools. For example, computers can be used to humanize or dehumanize medicine. The phrase "reproductive technology" is highly misleading and biased.

6. *Letting sensational cases skew our thinking:* When one case of commercial surrogacy goes awry, or when some "models" allegedly want to auction their eggs on the Internet, we incorrectly generalize to a thousand other cases where nothing similar occurs. So blinded are we by the media's extreme cases that we fail to heed normal rules of evidence, reason, and arithmetic.

7. *Ignoring the reality of mixed motives in people:* Most of us are neither saints nor villains. We are unlikely to donate bone marrow to strangers, and we are also unlikely to kill strangers. If public policy about organ donation, gene patenting, and parenting were to reflect this reality, we would have better results.

8. *Failing to note the opportunity cost of doing nothing:* When a new way of getting organs or offering reproductive assistance is discovered, opponents characteristically take a shotgun approach, throwing up every possible objection. Even if every objection is answered, the overall effect is a lingering sense that it is better not to change. Nowhere do people evaluate all the opportunity costs of being overly cautious and timid.

9. *Ignoring the role of money in discussing issues in bioethics:* Money may not make the world go 'round, but it is certainly worth paying attention to. Whether in medicine or academic biology, there are profound questions about the role of money almost everywhere, including biological research, assisted reproduction, and organ transplantation.

10. *In bioethics, failing to advocate positive changes:* Too many bioethicists are usually just naysayers: physician-assisted dying is wrong, human cloning is unthinkable, paying surrogate mothers exploits women, paying young women for their eggs destroys the family, germ-line genetic therapy is too dangerous, and allowing couples more choice about traits in children is eugenic. We are trained to be critical and condemnatory, not positive and supportive. Sometimes, bioethicists need to get behind and advocate new changes.

There are other mistakes people often make in discussing change in medical ethics, but the foregoing are the chief ones. I will discuss many examples of these mistakes in the rest of this book.

THIS BOOK IS DIFFERENT

I wrote a book in 1998 opposing some of the horrified reactions to human cloning.[3] In doing so, I was mindful of the lack of real thought in most people's gut reactions to that topic. I wrote this follow-up book because I find many of the same problems with many people's refusal to consider new ways of thinking about organ donation, reproductive help, computers in medicine, genetic choice, and bioethics.

Finally, the topics discussed in this book are in some sense unavoidable: they loom on the frontier of twenty-first-century medicine. As such, they pose the most exciting issues in journalism, health law, biology, medical sociology, and theology. The work here is almost all conceptual, and bioethicists are on the point, for we cannot look to the law or public policy, which are generally far behind. There is honest work here for bioethicists and others unafraid of entering new terrain.

True, risks abound in entering such unknown territory: one will be mistaken at times, either in fact or in judgment. So be it. But if you wait until all the new territory is explored and the maps are made, you are not participating in the discovery but following the course laid down by others.

NOTES

1. The talks were by Albert Jonsen and Dan Brock, respectively, on October 29 and 30, 1999, at the meeting of the American Society for Bioethics and Humanities in Philadelphia.

2. J. Marion Sims, *Uterine Surgery: With Special Reference to the Sterile Condition* (New York: William Wood, 1866), 361–70.

3. Gregory E. Pence, *Who's Afraid of Human Cloning?* (Lanham, Md.: Rowman & Littlefield, 1998).

2

RE-CREATING THE DOCTOR-PATIENT RELATIONSHIP: THE ETHICS OF CYBERMEDICINE

A growing number of patients, physicians, medical institutions, and businesses give and receive information via computers on the Internet. One recent survey found that more than 92 million adult Americans over age sixteen have used the Internet.[1] Roughly half of them have used the Internet to search for medical information.[2]

With so much information being exchanged so quickly, people can be both benefited and harmed. Little has been written to date about the *ethical* framework of such informational interchanges and about how it can be moral or immoral. This topic is important in the exploding fields of cybermedicine, medical informatics, telemedicine, health information technology, and clinical computing. Together, these fields fall under the category of cybermedicine, named after *Cybernetics*, the 1965 groundbreaking book by Norbert Wiener, and *Cybermedicine* by Warner Slack.[3]

What exemplifies immoral and moral informational frameworks in cybermedicine? Consider two examples. The first comes from a physician I know, call him David, a fiftyish white male internist in private practice in a city on the East Coast. One day while visiting with him, I brought up the topic of how patients are becoming more and more informed by reading *Consumer Reports*, the *New York Times'* Science Times section each Tuesday, and any of the many medical monthly newsletters, such as the one published by the Mayo Clinic. I also told him that, in researching the material for this chapter, I had discovered that patients were going on-line through the Internet, e-mail listservs, Yahoo, and AOL affinity groups to exchange information about diseases, physician responses, and drugs. "All in all," I exclaimed excitedly, "it is really empowering for patients."

David's response shocked me. He agreed with everything I said but found it quite threatening. In reaction, he told me he now subscribed to a special version of WebMD, a site only for physicians, and made patients fill out intake sheets before he saw them. He told me he had recently seen one patient in her sixties—call her "Mrs. Salzberg"—who had experienced a recurrence of polio. He knew little about such recurrences, but by having Mrs. Salzberg write her problem on her intake sheets, he had been able to *cheat* (his term) and look her symptoms up on WebMD. "By the time I let her come in five minutes later," he said, "I was the world's expert on recurrences of polio" (about which, by the way, little can be done).

I left this exchange feeling sad. Here was a physician who could have empowered his patient by telling her he didn't really know much about her problem but that *together* they could find out about it by searching the web. Instead of truly helping Mrs. Salzberg, David had harmed her by depriving her of an important fact ("I don't know any more about this condition than you do") and a more important tool ("but here is a way to learn everything about this condition and many other medical conditions"). By maintaining a false persona of omniscience, he had served his own needs but harmed hers. A more ego-secure physician, and perhaps, a less greedy one, would have been truthful with the patient about his own ignorance and would have helped her appreciate the Internet.

Some physicians would respond that there are patients who need their doctors to seem omniscient and that such an image is part of the art of healing. If so, tension exists between a patient's autonomy and her perceived best interest. Personally, I distrust such paternalism. In experimental surgery during the decades preceding the patient rights movement of the 1970s, therapeutic privilege was often abused when patients were denied information they needed in order to give real informed consent. Today, most patients get accurate information about life-threatening illnesses and are not harmed by getting it.

From the most general point of view, information is just a tool, and interactive-computer frameworks are in themselves morally neutral. It is the uses to which they are put, and the motives for doing so, that make them moral or immoral. Data are just data until someone decides to use them for some purpose; until then, data does not fall within the moral realm.[4]

Most of us would agree that harming people is immoral and, although in this case the harm done was slight and by omission, David's exchange with Mrs. Salzberg deliberately worked against her best interests.

Moral informational exchanges, ones that help and empower patients, rather than keep them in the position of passive children, do occur in cybermedicine. Such exchanges humanize both parties involved. What follows is an example of a moral exchange.

A fourth-year medical student named Sara had a sixteen-year-old patient named Anna who had recently been diagnosed with lupus and wouldn't take her medication (steroids), because they made her gain weight and made her face puffy. Anna's primary language was Spanish, and she spoke very little English. Even though she was tired from a long day's work at the hospital and wanted to go to sleep, Sara searched the Internet for a Spanish-speaking support group for teenagers with lupus. She eventually found such a group, based in California, and hooked Anna up with it. As Sara told me, "Now Anna's talking to other teenagers with lupus and sharing ways of dealing with her fellow classmates' teasing et cetera. I won't ever forget her. A real success story."[5]

In more ways than one. As a physician, Sara's compassion and orientation to patients is much different from David's. Sara not only helped her patient deal with lupus, she helped Anna initiate some friendships that may last for years. Sara didn't just give Anna a fish; she taught her how to fish.

These are two small examples and, in and of themselves, neither counts for much in the larger scheme of things. Nothing much can be done for recurrence of polio, and Anna probably would have eventually taken her steroids. But in a larger sense, when we consider the moral implications of how computers were used in these exchanges and how they can be repeated by many different physicians and patients, the direction a medical professional chooses to go makes a big difference, an *ethical* difference, to the kinds of relationships physicians will have with their patients.

I personally believe that something powerful is going on with Sara and Anna. Anna's entering into an on-line narrative with similarly diagnosed patients, especially when her physician has encouraged her to do so and is herself involved, not only encourages Anna to take her medication but also empowers her. Most importantly, the act *itself* could also *maximize healing*. Studies have shown that just keeping a narrative of one's life can be a powerful tool in healing.[6] At its best, cybermedicine creates and sustains just such a tool.

ENTER SKEPTICS

Skepticism about computers is not new. When I was in college during the 1960s, computers were regarded as evil machines used by Big Government to spy on patriotic citizens. The very image of a computer—a big mainframe spitting out hole-punched cards—was one of lurking menace. "One day," we said ominously to ourselves, "computers could run a dark world."

During those ignorant times, medical students needed a pass to enter the medical library, where the off-limits medical journals resided. It was important to keep patients and ordinary people out, because—poor children!—they might harm themselves by reading medical articles and drawing incorrect conclusions. The texts in the temple were only for the priests.

Many things changed all that. The advent of the personal computer made such machines an extension of a person's body and mind (the new designs of Macintosh's Imac, displayed in an array of vibrant colors, make them seem like kids' toys). Such personal tools have empowered people to write more, organize better, and express themselves more clearly. They have helped the disabled to function independently.

Laptops with wireless connections to the Internet extend a person's feeling of being connected, making a computer more like a cellular phone. Indeed, as miniaturization continues, Palm Pilots, cellular phones, and wireless laptops will likely merge into a wallet-sized device that will be phone, pager, E-mail source, Internet connection, and personal computer rolled into one.

For decades, computers have been connected across the planet (even before the existence of the web), but the computer also allowed *people* to connect with each other easily across the planet, preventing governments from being able to control their access to information. Far from being agents of governmental repression, PCs liberated people.

Originally, the Internet was built for the defense industry; gradually, academia and other institutions came on-line. The Internet was one of the few good things to come out of the paranoia of the Cold War, because it was built to be used as a safety net in case the Russians destroyed our phone system. At first, most people failed to understand the real implications of the Internet. Over the past decade, more and more information has been made public, even universal, on-line. As the cost of computers and scanners has dropped and as programs have been created to allow point-and-click creation of texts and pictures on web sites, the range of information available has increased dramatically. There was a time when a great story appeared in a city newspaper and disappeared the next day, having been read only by people in that city. Now a story can become immortal by being entered into the archives of the newspaper's web site and can be made accessible to anyone on the planet. Today, the web sites Medline and Grateful Med allow patients and physicians to access medical journal abstracts by pushing a few buttons on their home computers, and the *British Medical Journal* is completely on-line.

Even old folks eventually learned not to fear computers. For decades, my mother feared computers and the Internet. When she was seventy-five, her children got her a personal computer and connected her to E-mail. She and I now write back and forth more than we ever spoke on the phone—a phenomenon mirrored in the personal relationships of many other people that have been enhanced by E-mail. (Indeed, how many waning friendships have been thus saved? There's nothing quite like the surprise E-mail from someone you knew twenty years ago!)

As Andrew Shapiro writes in *The Control Revolution: How New Technology Is Putting Individuals in Charge and Changing the World We Know:*

> Before PC's became commonplace in the 1980s, most people thought of computers (if they thought of them at all) as mammoth objects with inscrutable vacuum tubes, blinking lights, and whirling magnetic tapes. This fearsome view of computers—straight from sci-fi movies and television shows—was abetted by the fact that these machines were scarcely seen in everyday life.[7]

For some people, computers symbolize technology and technology symbolizes what is bad about life. To these people, a computer is a machine that scares people, that replaces people, that substitutes dry facts for human emotions, and that calculates rather than intuits. Courses in philosophy of technology too often only focus on this negative sense of technology. As such, stories of replacing physicians by computers seem to exacerbate the dehumanization of both patients and physicians. No matter how good the program, no one wants to go into therapy with Dr. Feel Good, a computer therapist.

Some critics fear that doctors offices or HMOs will eventually substitute computers for avuncular, caring physicians. They fear that companies will use computers to reduce the time physicians spend interviewing patients (by having patients fill out interactive questionnaires in advance), thereby allowing physicians to squeeze more appointments into each hour.

Such critics fear that cybermedicine will create bad diagnoses by steering classified patients along preordained pathways and by using the myth of computer omniscience to create false impressions of scientific integrity. There is some evidence of this in so-called evidence-based guidelines used by some HMOs. These guidelines centralize diagnosis and treatment in a system, rather than in the physician–patient relationship, and hence, could harm individual patients.

One example of this is where computer programs such as the APACHE system are used to predict medical futility in end-of-life cases. Once a diagnosis of futility has been made, treatment could stop and death would be allowed to occur. Yet surely such an important judgment about a patient's death should reflect the particular details of the case, the personality and desires of the patient, and (presumably) a lifetime of experience of a consummate physician who brings all his wisdom, competence, and compassion to this ultimate decision.[8]

Moreover, many physicians believe that "outcomes research" by economists, health policy analysts, and HMOs is motivated by a desire to reduce the flexibility of physicians, curtail fee-for-service medicine, and give most patients what is merely good for patients rather than what is best. Outcomes research is almost always done via computers and by accessing databases containing patient records.

Such fears are not irrational. It should be stressed that computers and the Internet are morally neutral, just tools. It is the uses to which such tools are put that are moral or immoral. In the physician–patient relationship, the ethical question is whether such usage empowers physicians or empowers patients, or both. Computers and the Internet can certainly be used for bad purposes.

Richard Rockefeller, a pioneer of interactive cybermedicine with patients, argues that computers should be used to do the things that computers do well so physicians can get back to doing what physicians do well.[9] Computers can dehumanize or rehumanize medical care: the choice is each physician's, each clinic's, each medical system's. Cybermedicine can celebrate each patient's uniqueness, allowing him or her to tell personal stories and to monitor his or her evolving patient record. It can allow each patient to share his specific values, aversions, phobias, or tolerance for risk (as we shall see, allowing patients to accept some degree of risk will be a big theme of this book, especially of chapter 8).

Cybermedicine can bring up-to-date medical information to patients who are geographically isolated. It can be used by specialists to help primary care physicians in remote areas. Consider the Colusa County study of using telemedicine to monitor distant pregnancies, which followed expectant mothers in a county 60 miles north of Sacramento, California, where there were no obstetricians at the local clinic (forty-eight other of California's fifty-eight counties are partially or fully lacking such specialists).[10] Using telemedicine, obstetricians at the University of California at Davis Medical Center (UCDMC) followed expectant women and allowed 75 percent to deliver in their home county, whereas previously, all had to travel to a larger medical center outside their county. Similar projects in Australia allowed psychiatrists and nephrologists to assist patients in faraway towns.[11]

Another benefit for patients is ease of second opinions. Suppose you are in San Diego and are considering a risky facial operation for burn scars. It may also turn out that the best diagnostician is on the other side of the country (or globe). You go on-line and discover that the Orentreich Clinic in Manhattan has the most experience with operations that attempt to correct burn scars. Your California HMO will not pay for you to go to Manhattan or for Norman Orentreich to examine you, but as a compromise, you suggest a "telemedicine consult." Using live visual feeds from an Internet-II site, your second opinion is approved and Dr. Orentreich suggests some preoperative preparations that will maximize your chances of having a successful operation.

Cybermedicine can also achieve the great virtue of an ethical informational framework in that it can make the "how and why" of decisions about a patient's medical treatment *transparent* to everyone. Transparency fulfills what philosopher John Rawls champions as a virtue of just systems: their rules are open and public, allowing public discussion, accountability, and corrections.[12] It is not just the equal flow of information to both patient and physician that is important here, but the open, public nature of the flow. What is public and open can be critiqued, corrected, and made into a public good.

In an ideal informational framework, information does not flow to either physician or patient exclusively, but to both in a shared format. Joint decision making based on common, open information is the ideal arrangement of an ethical informational system. Shared decision making empowers and humanizes both patient and physician.

Practically and medically, many medical conditions, including benign enlarged prostate, low back pain, mild hypertension, benign uterine conditions, hormone replacement therapy, diabetes, depression, treatment for any kind of cancer or heart disease, and almost anything to do with birth control, assisted reproduction, or the dying process, are best managed through joint decision making.

Albert Mulley and others have tried to prove that shared decision making for some of these conditions results in greater efficiency, lower costs, better integration of nursing, less surgery, and more satisfied patients.[13] Nevertheless, proving that shared decision making reduces costs and leads to better outcomes is notoriously difficult. But such proofs about costs and clinical outcomes are peripheral to the main ethical point here: a shared, equal framework for information exchange treats physician and patient as moral equals in a common endeavor of healing. The reason shared decision making should be pursued in the use of computers in medicine and indeed in all of medicine is because of that ethical ideal, not primarily because of desires to save money or achieve better clinical outcomes.

Medicine really could be made simultaneously more ethical and more humanistic by using computers. As physician Atul Gawande writes in the March 1998 *New Yorker*, "As expert systems, both large institutions and microcomputers, begin to take on more of the technical and cognitive work of medicine, generalist physicians will be in a position to embrace the humanistic dimension of care. They'll be freed to do what only they can do—talk to their patients, for instance."[14] What computers are used for in medicine depends on the physician, not the computer.

One of the most astonishing things that computers can do in joint partnerships with physicians and patients is to aid both. In one recent Swedish study, a computerized program was pitted against a famous cardiologist in reading 240 EKGs of people, half of whom had experienced heart attacks. Reading EKGs to determine whether patients have suffered a heart attack is notoriously difficult to do. And in this medical version of the famous chess contest between the computer "Deep Blue" and Garry Kasparov, a different computer with a sophisticated medical program correctly diagnosed heart attacks 20 percent more accurately than the expert cardiologist (in other words, the expert either missed a real heart attack or made a false-positive diagnosis in 20 percent [24] of the cases).[15] Suddenly worries about computers dehumanizing medicine seem silly. Who *wouldn't* want this type of computer-assisted help for his cardiologist?

One specific worry about the physician–patient relationship concerns patients who are routed by computerized protocols to standardized treatment plans that ultimately fail. When such normal treatment fails, patients can be made to feel that they are economic "outliers" and, hence, aberrant, bothersome, and wanting treatment that is exorbitant. Again, how information technology is used depends on the motives of the designers of the system as well as on the consequences to patients. Patients with abnormal values should not be made to feel bad or be treated badly. After all, there is an old word for such patients: *ill.*

AN EXAMPLE: THE BRAIN-TUMOR SUPPORT GROUP ON-LINE

Computers and the Internet can be used in many creative ways to humanize physician–patient relationships. Consider the current situation for many patients. Few Americans have a general physician who cares for them from cradle to birth and who makes house calls. Few people have a physician who really *knows* them. Physicians' desires to earn a maximal income can cause them to double- and triple-book patients for the same twenty-minute slots, resulting in hurried interviews, long waits, and a needless waste of patients' time.

As strange as it may sound to some, computers and the Internet can help both physicians and patients to be more human. Consider the forty-year-old woman who suddenly experiences strange headaches, sees a physician, has a CAT scan, and is diagnosed with brain cancer. Can there be more frightening medical news? Once the words *brain cancer* have been said, the patient will hear little more of the conversation, as she tries to process that terrible bit of information.

Such a patient, let's call her Mary, a housewife on a farm near a small town in the middle of Iowa, feels immediately isolated from all other humans who don't have brain cancer, even her husband, parents, and her own children. *They* don't have brain cancer. *They* don't know what it feels like. *They* aren't going to die early.

Mary could be emotionally isolated whether she works a farm in the middle of Iowa or lives in a high-rise condominium in Manhattan's Upper East Side. In a short while, she will share her bad news with someone close to her. Most likely that person will be at a loss for words. More often than not, such patients report, people respond by saying nonthinking things like "I know just what you feel."

Mary will soon call her oncologist or neurosurgeon to ask further questions about possible outcomes and treatments. Almost always, this person, who is now her lifeline to information about her diagnosis and prognosis, was previously a stranger to her.

Modern life is full of horror stories about such patients being treated badly by the medical system. The character played by William Hurt in the movie *The Doctor*, a story about role-reversal when a physician gets cancer, powerfully portrays the pain experienced by a physician who is subjected to the treatment many cancer patients have been forced to endure.

That's the way it used to be, before patient-support groups began appearing on the Internet. Today, Mary can go to BRAINTMR, a listserv containing the names of people diagnosed with brain tumors and supportive nurses and physicians in this field, and hear stories of women in circumstances similar to her own.[16] Ideally, Mary's physician tells her about BRAINTMR, but she could also be told by one of her children or a friend or find out herself by searching on the Internet. BRAINTMR is probably by far the most important source of emotional support for people with brain tumors.

There are hundreds of groups offering such "life-support by E-mail." Groups exist that discuss the pros and cons of hysterectomies, natural childbirth planning, estrogen-replacement therapy, and new drugs for arthritis.

BRAINTMR was started by Samantha Jane Scolamiero in 1993. Three years earlier, Samantha had a brain tumor successfully removed, and afterward had problems with balance, clear thinking, and sensory overload. Because her tumor was benign, her insurance company wouldn't allow her to attend a nearby support group for people who had malignant tumors.[17] Alone and scared, she had difficulty getting her insurance company to pay for the best follow-up treatments and, even worse, had difficulty discovering what they were.

So she started BRAINTMR, an E-mail listserv that by 1997 had grown to twelve hundred members. This list has meant the difference between life and death for some members: "I doubt that what I say will come close to expressing the gratitude which I feel," one member wrote. "My sister would be dead today if it had not been for this support group."[18]

BRAINTMR contains personal narratives of patients who, faced with early death, must go to some very dark and frightening places of the soul. Such stories may not be what everyone wants to read, but they are invaluable for those who have been diagnosed similarly and who want to know that someone else feels exactly what they are feeling.

In another kind of case, when one woman's breast cancer recurred twelve years after successful treatment, she didn't want to burden her friends, so she went on-line to seek information. Her inquiries found sympathetic responses from the members of one chat group who called themselves "Cybersisters" and who easily persuaded her to join them. This woman's prognosis was still poor, but she says that her Cybersisters "have been extremely helpful to me."[19]

Patients find such electronic groups both comforting and empowering. Mary may find it too embarrassing to ask certain questions of her physicians: for example, whether a spouse will still want to have sex. Many patients find face-to-face revelations difficult but are able to reveal themselves anonymously on the Internet, which to some may serve as a confessional. Paradoxically, a person may be unable to reveal some personal intimate fact to three people sitting with her in a group, yet be able to tell the whole world the same information via the Internet.

There are reasons for this. With friends or relatives, roles and relationships have already been established, many of which may not be ideal support for patients. With the Internet, a woman who must stay at home with kids can read and post messages at anytime.

Undoubtedly, the greatest value of teaching patients about the Internet is to increase their autonomy and power to obtain maximal health. The Internet is ideal for patients with "orphan diseases"—diseases that are rare, not studied much, and not understood well by most physicians. It is also ideal for patients having conditions that might express a value preference not shared by most people. When Lisa Coles in Australia decided not to abort her fetus that had been diagnosed with spina bifida but to bring it to term, not many people would have agreed with her decision—but she found great support at the newsgroup site, alt.support.spina-bifida.[20]

Patients who are not afraid to be assertive and to ask questions can exercise autonomy on the Internet. A rheumatologist at one northeastern medical school told me about a woman who contacted him through E-mail concerning her fibromyalgia and gave him her medical history and lab data. The rheumatologist didn't like what he saw in the data and arranged to see her. He suspected that lung cancer was the real cause of her problems and that her previous physicians had attributed its signs to preexisting fibromyalgia. The woman was scanned, biopsied, and underwent surgery, having a 1.5-inch tumor with clear margins and no evidence of spreading metastasis excised from one of her lungs. A year later, she remained tumor free.

Two things had to happen to catch this cancer early. The patient had to be empowered to use the Internet and had to be bold enough to directly contact an expert over the Internet. The other is that the physician had to be open to responding.

Another woman, call her Patricia, who had diabetes, served herself well by being assertive on the Internet. Uncontrolled, diabetes can lead to blindness, a decrease in circulation, ultimately requiring amputation of limbs, and kidney failure. Patricia's non-insulin-dependent diabetes mellitus (type II) required monitoring her blood sugar levels and controlling her diet. Standard treatment didn't work well for her, and she went to a diabetes support group to learn better options. There, Patricia heard about a low carbohydrate diet that seemed right for her physically active mode of living, and she followed it successfully. She was irked to learn later that this option had been well known by her physician, who paternalistically had rejected it for her because of the diet's severe requirements (here was a case where shared decision making could have led to maximal health).

Postings of stories on listservs also create an electronic archive of the testimonials and struggles of the departed. Even at risk to their privacy, patients feel compelled to post the stories of their lives. As one patient on the BRAINTMR list says, "Someone has to SAY SOMETHING!"

Such networks allow sharing of information and end patients' isolation. They allow patients to be partners with their physicians in searching for information, rather than adversaries in a one-upmanship game. "At its best, the Internet elevates the patient–physician relationship into a partnership," claims Marvin Rorick, a doctor who claims to have been "humbled," but not ashamed, a few times when a patient could present more information about a condition "than I learned in medical school."[21]

Contrary to the fears of some doctors, patients such as Mary often gain greater faith in their physicians by participating in such groups. For example, undergoing certain treatments might seem very counterintuitive, but when other similar patients offer testimonials to the effectiveness of such treatments, initial skepticism turns to trust in the physician's recommendations.

Family members can use the lists to gain practical information, such as how to change a father's diapers or the fact that "magic mouthwash" cures the halitosis caused by many chemotherapies.

The BRAINTMR list humanizes physicians, as well, by showing them the inner lives and feelings of patients who have brain tumors. If any medical student ever needs a place to go to learn what it means to be diagnosed with a brain tumor, BRAINTMR is the place to go.

Today, support groups exist on the web for many diseases. The American Association of Cancer Online Resources (ACOR) moderates discussions of discussion groups under its auspices and censors flimflam postings. The University of Wisconsin at Madison sponsors CHESS, an on-line resource for cancer patients. The National Library of Medicine sponsors ASK-A-DOC, a service that lets people with cancer ask questions of nationally recognized oncologists and get answers within twenty-four hours.

MEDICAL INFORMATION: PATIENT LIBERATION OR PATIENT SERVITUDE?

"Knowledge is power," Francis Bacon said, and part of that knowledge is information. One of the unappreciated causes of the new, powerful U.S. economy is the accessibility of vast amounts of information through 120 cable television channels and the Internet and the fact that several national newspapers are available anywhere in the country.

But are patients participating in this new Information Age, or are they trapped as information serfs in some feudal setting? Who controls medical information about a patient: The patient? A physician? A hospital? The insurer? Medical information bureaus?

Questions about medical-information frameworks, in turn, are only a subset of a larger set of questions about the structuring of all such informational frameworks. Whether the relationship is one of business-seller, professor-student, pharmacist-client, or accountant-client, informational exchanges can be structured to harm or benefit those in positions of inferior power.

In the eighth century when Muslims fought Christians, the Moors conquered Gibraltar after already controlling Algeria and Morocco. By controlling this portal, Moor ships controlled the rich trade in spices and silks with the East. For the next five centuries, all trading ships that originated around the Mediterranean littoral paid the Moors.

Today, similar portals control what information people get. Some of these are ethical, some are not. In a famous paper, published in the *New England Journal of Medicine,* physician Mark Siegler argued that confidentiality today in medicine is a "decrepit concept," especially with electronic medical records.[22] Increasingly in the Information Age, control over information creates control over people. As Sheri Alpert concludes in her excellent review of the problem of confidentiality in medical-records computing, "Information has always been the lifeblood of business and industry. Those who control or influence the flow of information tend to thrive. This is no less true in the health professions and businesses."[23]

WHY PRIVACY MATTERS

In a moral framework, patients get maximal control over their medical information, which in turn gives them more control over their lives. Part of that control has to do with determining who does *not* see information about you. That kind of control is protected by the value of privacy.

As the philosopher James Rachels concludes, privacy is a good in general because it allows a person to control who has certain kinds of information about his life, which in turn allows him to control who he has relationships with and what kind of relationships they will be.[24] Sharing confidences is a prerequisite of intimacy, but one does not want to be intimate with everyone.[25] Controlling what happens to information about you by physicians is like controlling what happens to your body by physicians. In this sense, privacy enhances personal liberty.[26] As Thomas Nagel writes, we need to protect private life from "the crippling effects of the external gaze."[27]

Privacy is also important because we do not all share the same theory of the good (life). Although some thinkers write as if "the" theory of the good is discoverable, that is false. There are too many theories—from athletic body culture to sports fans who never exercise, from high achieving self-perfectionism to achievement-avoiding drug-dependency—for humans to ever accept one as "the" true one.

WHOSE CHART IS IT, ANYWAY?

In international affairs, we know that despots manipulate their citizens by controlling the information they receive on radio and television. China notoriously controls what the Chinese hear, for example, when the United States mistakenly bombed the Chinese embassy in Yugoslavia, China quickly manipulated its citizens into protesting in the streets (which it always banned in any context criticizing the government). Similarly, Slobodan Milosevic tried to control what Serbs felt and thought by controlling what they saw on television.[28]

As many others have remarked, the Internet, telephones, and faxes have subverted despotic control. Personal computers and the Internet are said to have brought down the communist Soviet Union, which could not both develop a communications infrastructure for a modern economy and also control information. When China shut down phone calls in and out of Tiananmen Square, faxes were used extensively to get news out. Until he shut it down, the B92 radio broadcasts from Serbia undermined Milosevic's control.

When it comes to medicine and democracy, is information more like dictatorships or more like going to a library? In medicine, there has always been a "Gibraltar" that a patient must negotiate to get information about his own body: the assumption that his medical records belong to the hospital or the physician, not him. But why continue a system built on that assumption? More important, why create new systems for the next century built on it?

Prima facie, information about a patient discovered by medical tests and physicians *should belong to the patient.* Her body and mind are the subject of the data, the data are of most concern to her, and in most cases, she paid for the tests that provided the data (at least indirectly, through paying insurance premiums). So why should her medical records reside exclusively in a hospital, or in a doctor's office?

Consider the fact that the average person moves every six years. Over a lifetime, a person may be seen by pediatricians, a general internist while in college, an assortment of physicians after college while getting a first job, another doctor after a big move or marriage, and an OB-GYN during pregnancy. Throughout these phases of her life, emergencies could occur—such as kidney stones, automobile accidents, injuries, and allergic reactions—which will not be entered into the cumulative medical record of any current physician she has. If she has a perfect memory and if everyone has the time, all her important past events will be revealed when a new physician takes her medical history—all very big assumptions! Given these facts, wouldn't it make more sense for the patient to have a copy of her own medical history that she could take with her, perhaps even encoded on a bracelet? With such a bracelet, paramedics could access a patient's medical records, find out any known allergies, and maximize on-the-spot treatment for injuries.

Suppose that after the birth of her first child she had a series of upper GI scans with radioactive dye, checking for a possible ulcer. Now twenty years later, she experiences the same problem and a new scan is done. Wouldn't it be good for her, and her physicians, to compare the two scans? Of course it would. Yet rarely is any effort made to find such previous records. (Yes, one can photocopy one's records, but as many people have experienced, it isn't easily done, and a request to do so may label one as a problem patient.)

So why isn't personal medical information readily available to patients? The answer goes back to Bacon: information is power, and in this case, the power is in control.

To see what a bizarre situation this is, consider how things would be if those in the business of repairing automobiles kept all the records and never gave any of them to the car owners. Suppose that your Toyota dealer kept all the records about your car, never giving you a copy of what the mechanic said, what was done to your car, or what price you paid for each service? Sounds silly, yet this is not too much different from what happens with medical records today.

Beginning in January 2000, UCLA Medical Center will spend $100 million to build a new hospital that will be easily accessible by anyone with proper authorization.[29] The digital system will be Internet-based and able to support information retrieval and input from many different clinical sites. Physicians will be able to write prescriptions, check lab results, and update a patient's chart—all via the Internet. According to the plans, using in-room web-TVs, patients will be able to order meals, track their treatment plans, and communicate with nurses and physicians.

But will they be able to access their own charts in these rooms? At home? Even physicians and nurses not involved in a patient's care will be able to call up a patient's chart to see what's going on. The sophisticated system, which will allow physicians to use personal palm devices to access the hospital's site on the Internet and, through it, patients' charts, might not allow patients similar access to their own charts while they sit in a room in the same hospital.

This is quite amazing, when you think about it. For one thing, there are real risks to patients when their medical records are made available on the Internet. In 1999, one HMO accidentally stored thousands of medical records on a public Internet site for two months.[30] Who knows who saw what while these records were posted? Second, consider that patients are always asked to consent to let insurance companies, employers, and government agencies see their medical records. As the former Office of Technology Assessment (OTA) noted in its report about privacy and computerized medical information, such inquisitive institutions commonly are the third-party payers, and since patients cannot otherwise pay for medical services, such consent seems to be indirectly coerced.[31] More important, if patients are not themselves customarily allowed to even see their records, how can they give *informed* consent to the release of those records to strangers?

Sure, there might be reasons for confidentiality when dealing with psychiatric patients, but for a gallbladder operation or heart surgery? Why does a patient's record concerning such interventions need to be hidden from her? Will computers be used to increase or decrease patient's access?

Of course, even getting one's chart is no panacea. Increasingly, charts are written in arcane language, understandable only to the "priest." Rather than "the patient has lung cancer," the entry will read "probable adeno-CA."[32]

These short-cuts have been taken to improve the efficiency of the hospital, for example by eliminating excess paperwork and medical records, instant filing of insurance claims, and immediate ability to track patterns in admission, testing, and mistakes. Not that these are bad things. In fact, some of them— greater efficiency and redundancy for patient protection—are in the patients' best interests.

I believe that this is the key point. Medical systems utilizing the Internet have to date been designed almost exclusively for physicians, not patients. Nevertheless, all is not lost, because the Internet is also the best available tool for reversing that trend. First, however, we have to admit it is a flaw in the present system.[33]

CYBERMEDICINE AND CONFIDENTIALITY

There are special dangers in computerizing patient files, in transferring information between computers, and in using Internet web sites as portals for physicians to enter medical data about patients. Confidentiality must be a central value in medical ethics, especially in the physician–patient relationship. Without an assurance of confidentiality, patients will not reveal personal sensitive information that is necessary for physicians to determine the best treatment. Confidentiality is not only important when patients want to control the spread of information about something "bad," such as having a sexually transmitted disease. Consider a woman who is the victim of a stalker and who doesn't want her address entered into the hospital's medical records (the stalker could be an employee of the hospital, who first saw her there).

At present, a patient's paper medical record in a hospital is one of the most nonconfidential, open documents anywhere, often hanging at the foot of a patient's bed or filed on a counter atop the nurses' station. Because it needs to be quickly available to anyone in case of emergency, it cannot be stored in a vault or locked up.

In the present circumstance, the number of people likely to be able to breach confidentiality, given minimal safeguards, is rather small compared with what could happen with electronic records. More than one person has inadvertently blurted out confidential medical information by mistakenly thinking he was replying to an individual on E-mail, when instead he was replying to a message sent by that individual to a listserv of thousands.

In any system, there are trade-offs between increasing confidentiality and other values. No system is totally confidential and protective against $50 thousand bribes to temporary employees. Any judgment about whether an informational system harms or helps patients, that is, whether it is immoral or moral, will involve how secure its information is from abuse by those who would harm patients. To increase confidentiality, several safeguards can be installed that will decrease the risk of leaks, such as limiting access to the system, using passwords, changing passwords every few months, and using encryption.

More generally, we need to ask for whom the system is designed. Is it designed in such a way that any physician, administrator, or head nurse can access the records of all patients? At a broader level, is it designed for access by residents, nurses, interns, and surgeons' assistants? Do the following need access: medical students, interns in hospital administration, nursing students, students in allied health? If anyone in a lab coat can access a patient's records, the system does not protect patients' privacy.

Confidentiality and privacy are values that cannot be absolute when the lives of others are at risk, but there are good and bad ways of breaking confidentiality. Consider the startling revelation that the San Francisco Health Department had traced an outbreak of syphilis to cyberspace.[34] This chat room was frequented by gay men in the San Francisco area who were looking for quick, semianonymous sex partners. This was the first case ever recorded of an Internet chat room being used for people to set up "outside" meetings to have sex, which resulted in them contracting a preventable, sexually transmitted disease. It was discovered that seven of the men using the chat room had contracted syphilis through unprotected sex and might be spreading it to other gay men.

Here is a case where the greatest good of the greatest number, or the public health, required a relaxation of strict privacy rights of individual members of America OnLine and members of this particular chat room. The case was handled deftly, as the San Francisco Department of Public Health persuaded a gay advocacy group to enter the chat room and post warnings. This falls far short of the "contact-tracing" method usually used by the Public Health Service, and it seems to have done the job.

Much of the previous discussion applies to the way in which the new Internet-II will work. It will be able to deliver not only words but images such as echocardiograms over special T-1 lines. In constructing this new network and in determining how patients and physicians will best be able to use it, it would be ideal to build confidentiality and security into the original design of the network rather than try to add it later. This is also true for the design of information systems in hospitals that serve physicians and patients. Doing so requires that patient-friendly values be implemented in the initial design.

At the end of 1999, President Clinton announced his intention to protect the privacy of electronic (not paper) records, but his plan would take two years to go into effect and anyone against the plan would have a chance to oppose it, so the net effect was unclear.

DATA AGGREGATION

There are businesses that exist to exploit health and sickness. For-profit medical insurance companies make the most money by insuring only healthy people, who make infrequent claims, and by refusing to issue policies to very sick people. In a world without a single-payer national medical system, U.S. Americans—unlike Canadians—could be at risk when they post personal medical stories on the net. When patients who have brain tumors post stories by name, information about them could be sold to companies seeking to hire only healthy employees. In 1999, President Clinton cited a survey of Fortune 500 companies that revealed that more than a third of them look at individual medical records before hiring or promoting employees.[35]

One example of an immoral informational framework was discovered by Laurel Simmons, the knowledge management officer at the Institute for Healthcare Improvement and founder/moderator of BMT-Talk (Bone Marrow Transplant Talk), a listserv with more than a thousand members for people who have had bone marrow transplants.[36] Simmons discovered a free portal funded by a group of businessmen and inviting people to sign on. In general, anyone who has a portal wants on-line users to use their portal as a home, so they can sell products with their banner ads. In this case, there were no banner ads, which aroused Laurel's suspicions. "How and why do they fund this expensive thing?" she wondered. "If they have no ads, how do they expect to make money?"

On their service, the businessmen promised confidentiality for people who signed on to their portals to obtain personalized access to all medical Internet sites. What the patients/clients didn't know is that they could have gone directly to these sites without going through this portal. It was like a real estate agent going through the newspaper apartment ads and charging people to show them apartments they could have seen on their own.

In this case, Simmons suspected the use of *data aggregation,* which is a technique for identifying a person and personal information about him without initially using his name or social security number. Way at the back of the agreement, about five clicks into the fine print, there was a message that said some of the data about the person—not his name or social security number—might be "aggregated" as group information and sold to commercial businesses.

One researcher, L. Sweeney, found that 80 percent of people can be uniquely identified from "de-identified" aggregated databases by using only the patient's birth date, zip code, and gender.[37] In a remarkable coup, this Massachusetts researcher uncovered the medical records of the governor of Massachusetts, William Weld. If a portal asks for and receives all of a person's E-mail addresses, it is much easier to identify that person and his medical records. This means that people should be wary of freely giving out their E-mail addresses, as more and more people ask for them, for example, on applications for bank cards or forms for magazine subscriptions: the more Venn diagrams that exist, the easier it is to discover the person on which they all intersect.[38]

Take Laurel Simmons's bone marrow transplant support group, BMT-Talk, for example. If people were required to go through a portal that did data aggregation to sign on to BMT-Talk, the company that owns that portal could identify 80 percent of the individuals on her mailing list, and identify them uniquely by name. Given the current incentives of employers not to hire employees with high medical risks, such unique identification is almost certainly not in the interest of citizens on the BMT-Talk list. Moreover, they would probably be under the false impression that they were anonymous and that companies needed their consent to identify them by name.

Many U.S. companies self-insure their employees, meaning that they create their own pool to cover their employees' medical costs. If such companies can hire employees of the same quality, but without any medical problems, they would make more money, because any unspent money from the workers' premiums would come back to the company. The 1993 report of the Office of Technology Assessment discovered a significant number of companies that will not hire people with serious preexisting medical conditions.[39]

There are private companies run by psychologists who interview prospective employees and give them a battery of personality tests. They charge hefty fees for their services and, if they do not tell management which employees to hire, they definitely tell them which employees *not* to hire. Are there now similar companies telling management which employees not to hire based on medical data aggregation?

Speaking of psychology and psychiatry, increasingly such records are being entered into remote sites, as HMOs badger psychotherapists for monthly and even weekly documentation as to why further treatment for a particular patient is necessary. The therapist must spend hours filling out forms and giving detailed information about diagnosis, treatment plans, medications taken (previously and presently), and past medical history. Frequently, in order to justify reimbursement, it might be necessary to make a condition sound worse than it is. And it is these dire diagnoses that get permanently entered into a record that could be "outed" one day.

Tipper Gore discovered something like this in 1999 as her husband announced his campaign to run for president and it was revealed that she had been treated for depression after the accidental death of one of her children. Obviously, talking to a therapist about such a death does not show mental illness (indeed, it probably shows mental health—ask yourself what it would mean if a parent *weren't* depressed after such a death?). The point is, it's become fair game to reveal the private medical records of anyone running for public office and anyone close to them. In 1972, the revelation that he had previously been treated with electroshock therapy for depression cost Senator Thomas Eagleton the Democratic Party's nomination for vice president.[40]

Breaches of confidentiality about sensitive personal information are surprisingly easy to come by. Many portals keep a record of the addresses of computers making inquiries, which can be linked to names of patients. Some inquiries immediately put the Internet user in special categories. For example, if a person makes an inquiry about where or how to test for HIV infection or where to buy an at-home HIV test, the inquiry might automatically place him in the group of people engaging in at-risk behavior (even if he is making the inquiry for his sister or a friend!). Suppose another person has no medical insurance, is self-employed, and has spent a lot of time recently talking with the on-line support group for those who have the gene for Huntington's disease. An insurance company that obtains such information might assume that he has tested positive for Huntington's or has a parent with this disease and hence, a 50 percent risk of inheriting it (although, again, he might just be doing a paper for a bioethics class!).

Information contained in medical records is not very well protected either. *New York Times* medical reporter Gina Kolata found that the medical records of Americans do not have much protection under federal law from companies wishing to buy information.[41] Some states, such as Alabama, offer patients almost no protection from third-party inquiries. On August 20, 1996, Congress gave itself three years to pass a bill protecting medical privacy. On August 20, 1999, it announced it had not met its deadline and "was still working on it."

MORAL AND IMMORAL PORTALS

The possibilities of data aggregation and breaches of confidentiality about sensitive personal information mean that some portals should not be trusted. Web sites that truly aim to help patients deserve the allegiance and loyalty of those patients, whereas those that try to sell goods to patients should be thought of in different terms, and those that attempt to sell information *about* patients (or deny them access to personal information) should be viewed in an even harsher light.

The Health Summit Working Group, composed of professionals in medical informatics and medical libraries, has for years been evaluating web sites that contain medical information.[42] The international members of this group adopted the following criteria, by which they judge whether a medical web site is moral: credibility, specification of which organization runs the site, frequency of updates, and whether medical experts have vetted the information available on the site. Also, a good site should contain layers of information, such that it directs the consumer-patient to sources of further information, such as sites at the National Library of Medicine or articles in medical journals via Grateful Med. Finally, according to the Health Summit Working Group, a good site should disclose whether it is collecting, using, or aggregating data provided by visitors to the site. It should also say who is funding the site (however, if ads are present, this might be obvious).

A portal's integrity is important because anyone or any company can post medical information. Sites run by firms selling alternative (a.k.a. "complementary") herbs and substances sometimes make claims that have no factual basis. In a 1999 study of 371 web sites with references to Ewing's sarcoma, a highly curable cancer, physicians found that 6 percent of the sites had serious errors, including one run by the *Encyclopaedia Britannica* (claiming the disease had a 95 percent mortality rate, even with radical therapy).[43]

Hospitals maintain web sites to supplement advertising and written brochures, all with the goal of recruiting patients. Such medical sites have a lot to lose financially if they provide false or misleading information. Nevertheless, in a 1998 study by pediatricians of web sites sponsored by major medical institutions, hospitals, and medical schools, it was found that 80 percent of such sites did not give the latest, best information about childhood diarrhea and in fact gave information that conflicted with the latest guidelines of the American Academy of Pediatrics.[44]

Perhaps the best sites and portals are run by agencies, advocacy groups, or organizations of patients linked by a common disease such as diabetes, cancer, or HIV.[45] However, not all sites that appear to be run by patients are in fact run by patients, and the information at any open discussion group or web site can be read by anyone.

CONCLUSIONS

The topic of the control of medical information and the uses to which it is put is a large and growing one. The surface has been barely scratched in this chapter.

Ethically, it is easy to draw conclusions about a system that helps patients rather than harms them. A moral system gives patients maximal control over commercial interests seeking access to their records. A hospital that makes money by selling such records is not in the business of promoting health, but in the business of making profits.

A patient should also have much more control than at present about who gets to see her record and should be able to readily see and obtain a copy of her own records.

The value of privacy and the confidentiality that protects it need to be rethought as we enter the age of cybermedicine. Privacy is crucial to some patients because it allows them to control their relationships with other people.

Our new age of computers, which are connected across the planet, brings new dangers to confidentiality: one physician blabbing at lunch might very well reveal something to an individual who shouldn't know, but a slip on the Internet can reveal such information to millions, making it immortal. We are now designing new systems in hospitals that contain such medical information, as well as the new Internet-II. Privacy and control of information about a patient should, in ethical systems, be built into the design from the start.

NOTES

I am very indebted to Laurel Simmons for her help with this chapter. Laurel founded and moderates the internet-based, Bone Marrow Transplantation Talk (BMT-Talk) and was a major presenter at a conference on cybermedicine sponsored by Harvard in May 1999.

In part, the idea for this chapter came from Neelaksh K. Varshney, a B.S./M.D. student of mine, whose 1998 seminar paper piqued my interest. This paper, "The Convergence of Medicine and Telecommunication: Implications for Patient Care," appears in the *Princeton Journal of Bioethics*, 2, no. 1 (Spring 1999): 18–32.

1. "92 Million Use Internet in North America," AP, *Birmingham News*, 18 June 1999, A11. Reports vary widely as to how many Americans either use the Internet or use it to find medical information. Jane Brody cites a figure of 22.5 million Americans ("Tips for Seeking Remedies on the Web," *New York Times*, 5 September 1999), whereas the

MSNBC link to HealthQuick.com says 18 million sought medical information. Undoubtedly some guesswork is going on here, but at any rate, millions of people are in fact using the Internet for this purpose.

2. Tom Ferguson, "Health Online and the Empowered Medical Consumer," *The Ferguson Report—The Newsletter of Consumer Health Informatics and Online Health* at doctom@doctom.com.

3. Norbert Wiener, *Cybernetics, or Communication and Control in the Animal* (Cambridge, Mass.: MIT Press, 1965); Warner Slack, *Cybermedicine: How Computing Empowers Doctors and Patients* (San Francisco: Jossey-Bass, 1997).

4. Sometimes, given known human motives and outcomes, it might be best not to acquire certain potentially dangerous data. We could test everyone in the country for HIV infection or presymptomatic genetic diseases and claim that we would just keep the information in a database to use for future comparisons and "look-back" studies. But it would be hard to keep the data confidential. Arguing from the best of motives, some would say that we need to identify those who are HIV infected and get them treatment and that it would be immoral not to break confidentiality in this case. If a technique became available to treat genetic diseases before they became symptomatic, similar arguments would apply.

5. Thanks to my former student Sara Helmbock, now a graduate of the University of Illinois Medical School, for sharing this story with me. The story is told with her permission.

6. Arthur Kleinman, *The Illness Narratives: Suffering, Healing, and the Human Condition* (New York: Basic Books, 1989).

7. Andrew Shapiro, *The Control Revolution: How New Technology Is Putting Individuals in Charge and Changing the World We Know* (Los Angeles: The Century Foundation, 1999 [www.controlrevolution.com]), 26.

8. I owe this point to Kenneth Goodman.

9. Richard Rockefeller, "The Interactive Computer in Patient Care," conference on cybermedicine, Harvard University, May 1999.

10. Telehealth/Telemedicine Coordination Project Report. Section 1 of home page. 5 January 1999, http://www.catehealth.org/secl.html.

11. "Discussion Papers on Telemedicine," John Mitchell and Associates, 24 October 1998, http://www.jma.com.au/telemed.html.

12. John Rawls, *A Theory of Justice* (Cambridge, Mass.: Harvard University Press, 1971).

13. Albert G. Mulley, "Improving the Quality of Decision Making," *Journal of Clinical Outcomes Management* 2, no. 1 (1995): 9–10.

14. Atul Gawande, "No Mistake," *New Yorker* (March 1998): 74–81.

15. Lars Edenbradnt and William Baxt, quoted by Atul Gawande, ibid.

16. *Listserv* is actually a trademark used for an Internet mailing list software written by a company called L-Soft. It has become a generic term for mailing list software, much like *Xerox* has become generic for photocopying.

17. Actually, the situation was even worse: Samantha was told *by the local support group* that she could not attend the group because her tumor was benign. Personal communication from Samantha Jane through Laurel Simmons.

18. Quoted by Dominic Gates, "Life Support by Email: Finding Help in a Medical Crisis," *PreText Magazine*, www.pretext.com/dec97/features/story1.htm (December 1997): Issue #3.

19. Ibid.

20. Ibid.

21. Quoted by George Court, "Web Medicine," Scripps-Howard News Service, *Birmingham Post-Herald*, 29 March 1999, D4.

22. Mark Siegler, "Confidentiality in Medicine: A Decrepit Concept," *New England Journal of Medicine* 307, no. 24 (9 December 1982): 1518–21.

23. Sheri A. Alpert, "Health Care Information: Access, Confidentiality, and Good Practice," in *Ethics, Computing, and Medicine*, ed. Kenneth W. Goodman (New York: Cambridge University Press, 1997), 92.

24. James Rachels, "Why Privacy Is Important," *Philosophy and Public Affairs* 4 (1975): 323–33; reprinted in *Can Ethics Provide Answers? and Other Essays in Moral Philosophy*, ed. James Rachels (Lanham, Md.: Rowman & Littlefield, 1997), 145–55.

25. I owe this point to Lisa Parker's talk at the ASBH meeting in October 1999, "Information(al) Matters: Broadening Bioethics."

26. Thanks to Laurel Simmons and Ted Benditt for helping me think about these points.

27. Thomas Nagel, "Concealment and Exposure," *Philosophy and Public Affairs*, 27, no. 1 (Winter 1998): 3–30.

28. The United States government also controls some kinds of information available to citizens, although usually in more subtle ways. The national media do the same, although more by follow-the-leader than by conspiracy. For years, stories about AIDS had a boom-or-bust cycle, with saturation coverage of a story for a few days, then nothing for months.

29. Mark Dwortzan, "Surf Your Prognosis!" *Technology Review* (May-June 1999): 29.

30. Mike Hudson, "Clinton Adds Rules on Medical Privacy," *Philadelphia Enquirer*, 30 October 1999, A3.

31. Office of Technology Assessment, *Protecting Privacy in Computerized Medical Information* (Washington, D.C.: GPO, 1993).

32. Perri Klass, *A Not Entirely Benign Procedure: Four Years as a Medical Student* (New York: Penguin/Plume, 1987), 76.

33. Laurel Simmons, personal communication, 7 October 1999.

34. Evelyn Nieves, "Privacy Questions Raised in Cases of Syphilis Linked to Chat Room," *New York Times*, 25 August 1999, A1, A16.

35. Mike Hudson, "Clinton Adds Rules," *USA Today*, 30 October 1999, A3.

36. This information is from a talk by Laurel Simmons, "The Internet and the Patient: What's Next?" at the conference on cybermedicine, Harvard University, May 1999. Quoted with her permission.

37. L. Sweeney, *Proceedings of the American Medical Informatics Association Fall Symposium*, 1997, 51–5. Laurel Simmons reports that this amazing result was duplicated at the MIT Laboratory for Computer Science.

38. Of course, it is possible to engage in moral Internet marketing, for example by explicitly seeking permission of potential consumers and by getting informed consent in advance regarding whom the information will be released to and why. Credit card companies ask permission of holders to sell information to marketing companies (and of course, some customers refuse).

39. Office of Technology Assessment, *Protecting Privacy in Computerized Medical Information* (September 1993). The OTA was abolished by Congress in 1995, but its reports are archived online by Princeton University at www.wws.princeton.edu/~ota.

40. "Eagleton Treated for Depression by ElectroShock," *New York Times*, 26 July 1972, A1.

41. Gina Kolata, "When Patient Records Are Commodities for Sale," *New York Times*, 15 November 1995, A1, B7.

42. Court, "Web Medicine," D4.

43. Jane Brody, "The Health Hazards of Point-and-Click Medicine," *New York Times*, 31 August 1999, D6. The study was led by J. Sybil Biermann and appeared in an August 1999 issue of *Cancer*: "Tips for Seeking Remedies on the Web," *New York Times*, 5 September 1999; reprinted in *Birmingham Post-Herald*, 6 September 1999, A5.

44. Brody, "The Health Hazards." The lead author was J. Juhling McClung, and the study was published in *Pediatrics*: "The Internet as a Source for Current Patient Information," *Pediatrics*, June 1998, 101.

45. According to Jane Brody's previously cited *New York Times* health columns, the following sites rely on information reviewed by peers of medical researchers and reports in reputable medical journals: Medscape, Healthfinder, Medhunt, National Institutes of Health, Centerwatch, National Library of Medicine, and Mayo Clinic.

3

RE-CREATING ORGAN DONATION: THE CASE FOR REIMBURSEMENT

He who saves a fellow creature from drowning does what is morally right, whether his motive be duty or the hope of being paid for his trouble.

—John Stuart Mill, *Utilitarianism*

In February 1999, famous NFL running back Walter Payton announced that he needed a liver transplant; he didn't get one and died that November.[1] In 1997, more than 1,130 Americans died while waiting for a matching liver. Yet there is a way to increase the donation of livers that we have never tried.

Physicians in 1954 witnessed the first kidney transplant at the Peter Bent Brigham Hospital in Boston, and since then, the demand for donated kidneys has far surpassed the supply. In 1967, Christiaan Barnard performed the first heart transplant in Cape Town, South Africa. In 1976, discovery of the antirejection drug cyclosporin A enabled some transplant recipients to live for decades. Years later, livers and lungs were also successfully transplanted. These surgical achievements caused the demand for organs to grow exponentially.

One of the great taboos in transplant medicine has been against the rational discussion of using financial incentives to increase the donation of organs for these life-saving transplants. Almost universally, transplant surgeons condemn this option. Some U.S. bioethicists have followed suit, claiming that "rewarded giving" is unethical.

I believe that it's time for financial incentives to be carefully considered. In this chapter, I discuss three ways in which such incentives might piggyback on altruism to increase the donation of organs. Many of the objections that arise here recur in chapter 4, where financial incentives for reproductive assistance are discussed. Read together, these two chapters reveal just how many human lives—both living and uncreated—are lost because of our reluctance to use financial incentives.

Our present system, lacking monetary incentives and with demand outpacing supply of organs, unsuccessfully tries to use the media to increase supply. But the media is more interested in controversial cases concerning just allocation. So we agonize over a prisoner who wants to donate a kidney to his daughter and query whether a fourteen-year-old boy from Wheaton, Maryland, should have received three quadruple organ transplants within nine months, including three livers.[2]

Instead of agonizing over how best to allocate what organs we have, we need to think about how to increase our supply. Sometimes, the way to solve the classic example of distributive justice, of who gets the rare dialysis machine, is to build a new factory.

To say that we need to think about using money to increase the supply of organs does not mean that we need to abruptly move from an altruistic, voluntary system to a crass, "anything goes" commercial system. Ethics is about drawing lines, and we might just be able to push up the supply of organs with only modest use of monetary incentives.

THREE METHODS OF REWARDING ORGAN TRANSFERS

Three general methods using monetary incentives could increase organ transfers. The first, and most controversial, is a *pure market system*, a system that could work only for kidneys, bone marrow, and possibly lobes of regenerable livers. This system would allow a competent adult to sell, for example, one of his kidneys to another person on an open market, where buyer and seller negotiate the price. The second is a *regulated system* where a mediating agency sets a uniform price and guarantees conditions on both sides, such as the informed consent of the seller and, for the buyer, the quality of the organ bought. The regulating agency could also pay the cost of acquiring the organ, so that wealth does not affect who receives the organ. The final system is *rewarded cadaveric donation*, which consists of paying families to encourage them to donate organs of brain-dead relatives (also known in medicine as "cadaveric donations").

In this debate, to date, the kidney has received the most attention for several reasons: it is sellable probably without harming the seller's long-term health; it was successfully transplanted before hearts and livers; and it has a backup when its transplantation fails (since 1962, when the creation of the in-dwelling shunt allowed long-term hemodialysis).

In India, a desperate situation helped create a pure market in organs among competent adults. Among many Hindus, beliefs about caste and karma, as well as desires to cremate the entire body and set it adrift in the Ganges, make families unlikely to consent to cadaveric donation. Meanwhile, as many as eighty thousand Indians each year experience end-stage renal failure, while only 650 dialysis machines exist in the country.[3] Without a kidney transplant, many of these eighty thousand Indians will die.

This dire need created a system whereby healthy Indians could sell one of their kidneys. About two thousand Indians did so each year, where buyers paid $6 thousand to $10 thousand and the seller got about $1 thousand.[4]

Such a pure market system seems repugnant to most people, in part because it allows a competent adult to risk harm to himself. But we should remember that people may *donate* kidneys to others and risk exactly the same harm to themselves. Frequently praised in the national media, no one questions whether altruistic, living donors are sane, being exploited, or making bad decisions. Thus, what is morally objectionable cannot be the possible harm to a competent adult transferring one of his kidneys to another.

What must make a pure market system objectionable has to be the exchange of money. But this objection is odd when we look to human nature and compare motivations. People are allowed to risk harm to themselves for pure altruism, but they are not allowed to do so for a million dollars. People are now allowed to sell their time, knowledge, and the best years of their lives to employers. In the United States, people are at present allowed to sell their sperm, eggs, hair, blood, and cadaver.

Richard Epstein, a libertarian professor of law at the University of Chicago, argues that advantages of the pure market system include the fact that the transplant can be timed under optimal conditions and with optimal matches.[5] With the luxury of time, no dramatic helicopter rides, or sprints with iced organs in Igloo containers, need occur.[6] Nor is there the "multiple veto problem" that occurs with the other cadaveric system, where family members can veto the decision of a deceased, previously competent adult to donate an organ.

The third system, rewarded cadaveric donation, is now under consideration in Pennsylvania, which is the home of Pittsburgh's famous transplant program. The state has proposed paying families $300 toward funeral expenses, with the plan funded through fees for driver's licenses.[7] Under this method, all families get the same payment and organs are distributed to the most needy. Thus, the plan has no real market, only a monetary payment to encourage donation, so this is also a regulated system.

Whereas the pure market system applies only to a few body parts, rewarded cadaveric donation generates hearts and lungs, bone marrow, skin, corneas, and the body itself.

BACKGROUND: REIMBURSING FOR HUMAN ORGANS

Obviously, the possible exchange of money in organ transfers creates a lot of moral concern, and because every moral issue has a pedigree, the history of this concern is enlightening.

Sometimes in U.S. medicine, the public first hears about a good idea under the worst of circumstances, for example, when an idea is first espoused by a famous eccentric. Such death by association came when Jack Kevorkian publicly supported physician-assisted dying ("Kevorking" the issue) and when Chicago physicist Richard Seed announced he wanted to clone himself ("Seeding" the issue).

The earliest blow to the rational consideration of paid organ donation may have come from the controversial origins in the United States of paid *blood* donation, a system begun by a similar eccentric. Francis H. Bass, a former used-car salesman, started the first commercial blood bank in 1955 as a way to make a lot of money for himself.[8] His blood bank battled nonprofit, hospital-based blood banks, which took the moral high road that all donation of blood should be unpaid. The hospitals refused to do business with Bass, but he sued them and won when the Federal Trade Commission ruled in 1964 that the hospitals were in violation of free trade.[9]

Nevertheless, the idea of paying for blood never transcended its eccentric origins. Had a distinguished physician and a proper hospital proposed to pay for blood, things might have been different.

The fatal blow to paid organ donation came from another person in this undistinguished line, businessman H. Barry Jacobs of Virginia. In 1983, Jacobs announced plans to start International Kidney Exchange, Ltd., an organization through which competent adults could buy and sell kidneys.[10] The abhorrent part was that he planned on using indigent immigrants as sources for his organs.

At the time, such a business was not illegal in Virginia or in the United States, and Jacobs announced that his brokerage fees would make his operation "a very lucrative business."[11] Jacobs's proposed business, and the way he talked about it, painted a morally repugnant picture: affluent people buying the kidneys of desperately poor people recently arrived in the United States, with unscrupulous brokers pocketing huge fees.

In reaction, a House subcommittee chaired by Albert Gore held hearings and recommended criminalizing the sale of organs; Congress soon followed its recommendation. Monetary incentives for organ donation became illegal, a violation of federal law, under the National Organ Transplantation Act of 1984, punishable by ten years in prison and a $500 thousand fine.

The 1971 publication of Kenneth Titmuss's *The Gift Relationship: From Human Blood to Social Policy* had previously dealt another blow to the impartial discussion of financial incentives for organ donation. Titmuss, an English sociology professor, disliked many aspects of American life. Parts of his 1968 book, *Commitment to Welfare*, spelled out this scorn with a vengeance. This book lambasted the U.S. medical system, which Titmuss saw as evil compared with the good, free, National Health Service, which—at least in theory and in those good old days—provided free, equal medical coverage for all English citizens.

Titmuss could not understand how any system with financial incentives and co-payments could be good, nor could he envisage the English system ever being inferior to the American system. In Titmuss's opinion, desires for profits corrupted the U.S. medical system, and U.S. physicians made obscene incomes, especially the overabundant specialists.

Indeed, writing in 1968, Titmuss implied that the U.S. medical system was on the verge of collapse, claiming shoddy education of physicians, too much self-diagnosis and self-referrals by patients to expensive, self-serving specialists (without the intermediary of the good English, family-physician-gatekeeper), and overbuilt, coast-to-coast hospital chains spread out like convenience stores to maximize profits. He predicted that such an out-of-control system would create unnecessary surgery/hospitalization and spiraling malpractice suits that would eventually cripple U.S. medicine.

So it was no surprise that his follow-up book, *The Gift Relationship*, expressed the same scorn and was meant to be a reductio ad absurdum of the American way of collecting blood. As Titmuss painted it, the contrast seemed stark and obvious: Americans bought blood from money-seeking alcoholics and prisoners, both of whom often carried blood-borne diseases and who were motivated to lie. In contrast, the altruistic English lined up good-naturedly and rolled up their sleeves for the needy. English blood was pure and free; American blood was dirty and bought. Need one say there was symbolism here?

As Douglas Starr observes in his masterful book on the history of blood, "Titmuss's book hit a public nerve. It generated scores of reviews in the news media and scholarly journals. It created a ripple effect. . . . The public now saw [as sources of American blood] the derelict and the prisoner."[12]

Titmuss's book conveyed the residual impression that Americans had erred by allowing blood to be commercialized. Given such an impression, it was unlikely that organ donation ever had any real chance of being similarly commercialized. There was a big battle here between good and evil. We had messed up once by choosing evil, and we certainly shouldn't choose that side again.

Alas, Titmuss never revealed the fact that the English never got enough blood through altruistic donation and had to buy blood from the United States. The English learned this painful fact in the 1980s, after imported American blood infected many surgical patients there with HIV infections.

In the early 1970s, when plasmapheresis was invented, which was very time-consuming but allowed much more frequent donation, few citizens anywhere underwent it altruistically. Almost universally, plasma donors had to be paid. In real life, altruism quickly finds it limits, so collection of plasma soon relied exclusively on paid donors, with U.S. firms exporting it to the world (and filling most of England's need for plasma).[13]

As noted in the introductory chapter, some ethical issues in medicine are conceptualized in simplistic extremes. With organ donation, we usually think this way: either a system is altruistic or profit-maximizing, which is like claiming that a physician must be either a missionary or a capitalist.

Life and medicine defy such simplistic categories. People have complex motives—some good, some bad. Systems have advantages and disadvantages. Painting a system with only one color prevents us from seeing the range of colors underneath.

For example, one of Titmuss's factual premises turned out to be false. He assumed that scientific technology would never be able to detect HIV or hepatitis C and, hence, blood collection would always need truthful donors. But tests now screen donated blood for the known strains of HIV and the known forms of hepatitis.[14]

Titmuss also implied that paying people would actually *reduce* altruistic giving. People who would have given altruistically would be demoralized by knowing that other people were being paid for blood. If that were really true, it would augur poorly for paying for organs. Yet Titmuss almost certainly *under*estimated the extent to which good business depends on moral values, but *over*estimated the strength of anonymous altruism in humans. Taken together, these faults led him to ignore the practical virtues of a mixed system.

As a result of the controversial history of commercial blood banks, of Barry Jacobs's plans, of Titmuss's work, and of an uncritical hostility toward commercialism in obtaining organs, Western transplant surgeons have always opposed financial incentives. In 1985, the Committee on Morals and Ethics of the Transplantation Society, believing it had to take a strong stand against inchoate commerce in kidneys, denounced the buying or selling of organs.[15] In 1985, 1987, and again in 1994, the World Medical Association condemned the purchase and sale of human organs.[16] In 1986 in the United States, the Organ Task

Force asserted that organs are the property of the "community," not of individuals to sell.

ARGUMENTS FOR REWARDED DONATION: SAVING LIVES

What is the strongest argument for rewarded organ donation? The answer is a direct one, appealing to life itself and not simply to indirect benefits. It's quite simple: doing so would save many lives. More than three thousand Americans die each year while waiting for an organ transplant that never occurs.[17] But it's not clear that this has to happen.

At this moment, more than eleven thousand Americans are becoming jaundiced while waiting for a donated liver. Every year since 1998, one thousand of these people have died. Another four thousand Americans are turning ash-gray from failing circulation, as they wait for a heart. During the 1990s, 750 or more people died each year awaiting a heart transplant.[18] By the end of 2000, more than forty thousand Americans will have died since 1988 awaiting an organ transplant (see table 3.1).[19]

So year after year, thousands of people die unnecessarily. Medicine has the scientific capacity, the facilities, and the personnel to save them, but the taboo against rewarded donation prevents it from doing so.

In reviewing past discussions of paid organ transfer, I am struck by the fact that no one on either side emphasizes the huge numbers of lives lost as a result of not permitting financial incentives for organ donation. Indeed, this loss is sometimes treated by opponents of financial incentives as almost mundane, as if it should be obvious that thousands of lives *must* be sacrificed on the altar of a non-coarsened social life.

Table 3.1   Patients Removed from the OPTN Waiting List Because of Death

Organ	1988	1989	1990	1991	1992	1993	1994	1995	1996	1997	1998
Heart/lung	61	74	66	41	43	51	47	28	49	56	41
Heart	493	517	613	778	779	761	724	769	745	772	767
Intestine	0	0	0	0	0	3	15	19	21	41	45
Kidney	734	749	916	974	1,047	1,777	1,365	1,503	1,802	1,989	2,295
Kidney/Pancreas	0	0	0	0	14	59	70	84	01	121	93
Liver	196	282	317	435	495	560	655	797	956	1,130	1,319
Lung	16	38	50	137	218	251	286	340	386	409	486
Pancreas	5	21	19	35	32	2	8	3	3	11	9
Overall	**1,494**	**1,659**	**1,958**	**2,351**	**2,573**	**2,883**	**3,053**	**3,414**	**3,896**	**4,313**	**4,855**

Source: United Network for Organ Sharing (UNOS), www.unos.org/newsroom/critdata_wait.htm.
Notes: Totals for each column will not equal overall total because some patients were listed more than once.

It is impossible to overemphasize the good that is being lost here. It is very immediate, tangible, and direct. It is the good of life itself, something that everyone believes is worth saving. Not only is saving lives an intrinsically good thing, but it is a morally commendable goal, against which few other goals stack up.

Life is precious. To allow it to be wasted, when simple changes in our medical-legal system could save it, is a tragedy of human making, not of divine fact. True, we didn't cause the diseases that destroyed the organs, but we continue to allow the system to operate that prevents lives from being saved. Even if we changed the system to allow only rewarded cadaveric donation, many lives would be saved. (Perhaps this is the only change we need to make for a few years, while we acquire data on how the change works and study unanticipated consequences.)

One of the great problems of ethics is to make judgments between "incommensurable" values. On the negative side, there is a risk of coarsening society by allowing financial incentives and also by giving up on the high ideal of widespread, altruistic donation. On the other side, there is the richness, creativity, beauty, and wonder of the human lives needlessly wasted. The number of such lives lost each year—whether we're talking about three thousand American lives or fifty thousand lives lost worldwide—must count very powerfully in any moral calculus.

Indeed, in any moral framework that emphasizes consequences to humans, for any competing value to be strong enough to trump this value, *it would have to involve an equal number of human lives saved or lost.*[20] But we are not in the situation here of philosopher Judith Thomson's famous trolley car example, where the driver of a runaway trolley car has the choice of diverting the train to the left and hitting two people or to the right and hitting a dozen.[21] Our situation is more like the one where there are a hundred people on the right and an empty, magnificent morgue on the left.

The great good of saving thousands of lives would be accompanied by indirect goods. Thousands of family members would continue to value the people saved. Some patients could continue working, paying premiums for medical plans and taxes and contributing to the economy and toward the costs of their

Table 3.2   Average Number of Organs from Cadavers (brain-dead patients), 1988–1993

Organ	Number Actually Acquired	Number Potentially Acquirable
Kidneys	8,000	18,000
Liver	3,000	7,000
Heart	2,000	6,000

Source: Author's estimates after talking to UNOS.

transplant. Families who received payment for cadaveric donation would at least get something out of the death, perhaps helping to pay for the education of their children.

Not only would monetary incentives increase the quantity of lives saved, they would also increase the quality of life of those living in wait for a transplant. There are currently eighty thousand people on dialysis in the United States, but fewer than 10 percent of them are listed as "clinically suitable" for kidney transplants. Many more would be listed, were donations to grow tenfold, and life with a new kidney would be far better for almost everyone than the tedious procedure of dialysis. Not only that, one study suggests that in the long run, it is cheaper to provide people with transplants than to keep them on dialysis.[22]

From a utilitarian point of view, where the number of people affected and the consequences matter, offering payment to families for cadaveric donation increases both the number of lives saved and the quality of life lived for those getting transplants. Many of the consequences of offering payment are positive. Using this theory, it is only rational that we should, at the very least, begin an experiment in a few states to see if rewarded cadaveric donation works to save lives.

INCENTIVES CREATE CHOICES, THEY DON'T COERCE THEM

Let us consider some indirect arguments in favor of financial incentives. Nearly thirty years ago when Titmuss's book was in vogue, Titmuss wrote that Americans were "coerced and constrained" by the option of being paid for their blood. Titmuss's claim was challenged by economist Kenneth Arrow, who declared that "creation of a market increases the individual's area of choice [and] therefore leads to higher benefits."[23]

This is an important debate for the rest of this book. It is common for both social liberals and social conservatives to see financial incentives as bad things for people, as making commodities of people's choices, their lives, and their bodies. They see systems that allow choices in terms of money—specifically in the buying and selling of things and the resulting prices being set by supply and demand—as coercive and exploitative.

Certainly there is a strong moral objection to such markets being created between individual competent adults, because inevitably some person somewhere who donated a kidney or part of his lung or liver would eventually die young. Or the operation itself might be iatrogenically lethal for the donor. Many people find it distasteful to envision people selling parts of themselves for money, although this seems more of an aesthetic objection than a moral one.

Similar objections do not apply to financial incentives to increase organ donation in a regulated system to pay family members to consent to donate organs from the bodies of brain-dead patients (especially here because the money never results in the death of an otherwise healthy patient). Nevertheless, many transplant surgeons seem to be against use of such incentives.

There is evidence that as a result of paying commissions to organ procurement officers and helping families pay for burial costs in exchange for cadaveric donations, Spaniards have gone from having the lowest to the highest organ donation rates in Europe.[24] People are motivated in part by self-interest and, in market economies, in part by money. That is not to say that people are *only* motivated by money or that everything should be allocated by markets. But money does affect human behavior. That this is true with organ donations can be seen in a more striking way by imagining what would happen if families were *charged*, say, one thousand dollars for each organ they donated. Would this have an effect on the number of families consenting to donate organs? (It appears so. Alabamians have expressed shock at the recent decision at my medical school to *charge* donors $750 for each body donated.)

Richard Epstein argues that infusing cash into organ transfers does not eliminate altruism but *refocuses* it to more appropriate targets. His real question is, "Who should be the altruist?" in organ transfers. The present system works the wrong way because, "Those who should be recipients of charity are asked in the name of altruism to sacrifice a second time, often for some nameless person."[25] But if payment were allowed, the burden would fall on taxpayers (if government offered cash incentives), not on the bereaved family.

ALTERNATIVES HAVEN'T WORKED

Lack of transplantable organs motivates surgeons to find ways around current limitations imposed by ethics and will continue to do so until there are enough organs. Like a flooding river, this urgent need keeps trying to find ways over, under, or around the various ethical dams that appear in its path. Consider the following three alternatives to offering financial incentives, all of which raise ethical problems, some more serious than those raised by the financial incentives we are considering.

First, proposals constantly surface to broaden the scope of eligible cadaveric donors. Most have failed, but surgeons keep trying to expand definitions of *dead person, nonperson,* and *never a person* to include young patients in persistent vegetative states, non-heart-beating donors (the controversial protocol originated at the University of Pittsburgh Medical Center, the transplant capital of the world), and anencephalic babies.[26] Such changes in definition, generally practiced out of the light of public scrutiny and certainly without real public understanding, only increase public distrust of the transplant system.

Second, dying people who need transplantable organs are constantly promised that breakthroughs are coming in artificial hearts, xenografts, and tissue engineering. A little perspective helps evaluate those claims. For example, surgeon Christiaan Barnard predicted in 1968 that pig hearts would be routinely transplanted into humans within twenty years.[27] Thirty-two years later, we are not much closer to performing such transplants, much less performing them "routinely." The artificial heart was a disaster, in some cases not even fitting into the empty cavity of the patient awaiting it.[28] Almost fifteen years later, no breakthroughs have occurred to solve the essential medical problems that plagued such devices. And where tissue engineering has done a good job of producing skin and ears, producing a functional heart or liver is another matter.

Third, proposals abound to get around the problem of families of brain-dead patients refusing to give voluntary, informed consent for donation. These proposals include required request (the law in most states, applying to families of potential cadaveric donors) and mandated choice (required request of individuals before they become potential donors, e.g., when they renew driver's licenses). When tried, such proposals have not increased the frequency of organ donation.

At worse, some proposals to change the system are unethical. Consider *presumed consent*, tried in Europe, where laws presume citizens consent to be organ donors, unless they state otherwise. Why has such a system failed and been considered immoral?

> the European model of "presumed consent" . . . is fundamentally dishonest. Under this regime the decedent or his next of kin have the legal right and theoretical power to opt out of donation but no clear mechanism with which to do so. Absent a national recording scheme, the decedent himself will almost never have an occasion to make his wishes known to the authorities. And, even his next of kin may be unaware of their right to choose on his behalf, or when that choice arises, or how to make their wishes known.[29]

Systems of presumed consent have failed to increase organ donation in Europe, and justifiably so. Most people believe that they have a property right in their bodies and that consent is necessary for the disposal of it. The law in some European countries allows physicians to simply commandeer organs without asking for consent of families, but most such physicians refuse to do so.

Fourth, and most important, at one time there was a ban on organ donations from living people, because of the traditional rule of medical ethics, *primum non nocere* ("first do no harm"). A surgeon who cuts part of the liver from a healthy person unequivocally harms the donor, and no matter how much medical professionals brush over the risks, there are indeed real, possible complications: unexpected reactions to anesthesia, iatrogenic infections, and even surgical accidents.

Consider the first transplant of a liver lobe from a live parent (a mother) to a daughter—Alyssa Smith. While he was removing the lobe of the donor's liver, the surgeon—Christopher Broelsch at the University of Chicago—nicked the mother's spleen and was forced to excise it. Broelsch called the loss of the donor's spleen a "major complication" and said that it gave him "the sickest feeling to have trouble with the first patient."[30] Undoubtedly, Broelsch's "sickest feeling" came from the inescapable knowledge that, in trying to help the sick daughter, he had injured the healthy mother.

The *primum non nocere ban* was broken with the first kidney transplant from one twin to another. The breaking of the rule was justified by the argument that the two identical twins were so close that the death of one would traumatize the other forever, especially if the one alive could have saved the other merely by giving up one of his two kidneys (the kidney was also a perfect match, assuring a high chance of success).

In another case in July 1993, Nilza Rodriguez gave one-quarter of her liver to her dying granddaughter. The prognosis for this donor was that her own liver would regrow and be perfectly normal "within a month or so."[31] In January 1993, in a precedent-setting case, fifty-five-year-old James Sewell and forty-nine-year-old Barbara Sewell each donated part of a lung to their twenty-two-year-old daughter, whose own lungs had been damaged by cystic fibrosis, a genetic disease that is typically fatal by age thirty. Adults dying of cystic fibrosis who get a lung transplant get a lung that doesn't create the mucous characteristic of this disease, so the patient no longer has cystic fibrosis and only has to worry about rejection. The Sewell case opened the door to a wave of such lung lobe transplants for teenagers with cystic fibrosis. By 1997, Vaughn Starnes had taken lobes from seventy-six donors for thirty-seven recipients. In the same year, one commentator noted that the practice was "ethically problematic."[32]

The probes of surgeons into this problematic, ethical territory make one wonder whether some questions should never be asked. We recognize that society must encourage heroes and saints, but routinely assuming that every parent will become a hero or a saint is a different matter. Is it fair to put parents in a situation where they are not just asked but *expected* to be saintly because of love for their children? Sure, parents can technically refuse, but virtually no parent does. Even the most loving parents must feel torn when considering donation to a dying child, yet how can they refuse something that could extend the child's life?

From a few isolated cases in 1993–1994, such requests are becoming the norm and even expected as the year 2000 begins: "There now exists an ethical imperative to develop this [live-donor donation of livers]," says Jean Emond, director of liver transplantation at New York Presbyterian Hospital in a September 1999 *American Medical News* front-page story.[33] Adult-to-children liver transplants require a small portion of the adult's liver. Adult-to-adult liver transplants require a higher percentage of the liver to be transplanted, usually the entire right lobe, or 60 percent of the donor's liver function, creating more risk. Nevertheless, seventy adult living-related transplants were performed over the past three years, with forty-five in the first half of 1999, showing the exponential growth. In September 1999, the first death from adult-to-adult liver donation was "confirmed," although not "officially described" (probably in order not to dampen enthusiasm for this new source of organs), and it was reported that about two to three adults are estimated to have died from donating parts of organs to their children.[34]

As I shall stress shortly, I am not arguing that such requests are unethical. Rather, I cite this problem and others to emphasize the extremes to which we go in our present system, without financial incentives, to increase available organs. All three of the general methods discussed for increasing the supply of organs—redefining death, changing consent, and taking organs from healthy relatives—raise enormous ethical problems for all involved and for public policy.

I have stressed that much of the transplant ethics involves a false "first step," where only two simplistic alternatives are discussed, with the implication that one is pure, the other, base. The alternative of some mixed system, for example, rewarded cadaveric donation, needs to be a viable alternative that gets consideration.

The messy ethical dilemmas raised by the three issues discussed previously show that our present system has many problems. Second, and somewhat extraordinarily, *rather than paying families for organs from cadavers, we are asking some members of families to be live donors and in the process, unintentionally killing some of them.* Some parents who entered the hospital healthy left it dead.

And the problems are growing. Last year, more than four thousand living donors gave kidneys to relatives, life partners, or someone they knew, and one hundred people similarly gave part of their livers.[35] Moreover, in a bizarre new twist, two Good Samaritans have now approached a hospital, wanting to give up a kidney to no one in particular, just willing to do so. They were accepted and one of their kidneys was removed.[36]

Are such people competent to do this? Altruism is wonderful, but do we uncritically accept this new development while still claiming that rewarded cadaveric donation is unthinkable?

Moreover, one of the primary objections against a regulated system of financial incentives between competent adults for organ transfers is the possible deaths of otherwise healthy donors. But precisely the same harm is now permitted by the present system to obtain more organs by encouraging live donors to consent to transplantation! How can this be consistent?

Finally, note that the present system of presumed altruism doesn't work for people who are uncomfortable asking a relative or spouse to donate a kidney but who would be comfortable receiving a kidney from a family paid to donate it from a cadaver. Also, just because no compensation takes place does not mean there is no pressure or coercion (there are cases of coerced donations from wives to Indian husbands in renal failure). One can also imagine great pressure within a family (say, with identical twins) to donate.

HYPOCRITICAL AND INCONSISTENT

American medicine makes very few transplants available free to those without medical coverage, so it is hypocritical to maintain that our present system is not influenced by money. Isn't it also hypocritical that the only people *not* paid in the whole system of organ transplantation are the families of donors? Everyone else gets paid, and paid very well indeed. As the Bellagio Report on paid organ transplantation observed in 1997, "After-all, transplantation is hardly a commercial-free transaction. Hospitals, surgeons, organ retrieval teams and procurement organizations regularly sell their services. Why should the source of the organ be the only one not financially rewarded?"[37]

As I said before, blood, eggs, semen, tissue, spines, and entire cadavers are already being sold. Why not then allow payment for kidneys from cadavers? As the Bellagio Report concluded in 1997:

> the sale of body parts is already so widespread that it is not self-evident why solid organs should be excluded. In many countries, blood, sperm, and ova may be sold. So too, an international trade exists in cadaveric body parts for medical education and research, and pharmaceutical companies purchase large quantities of tissue for commercial purposes. Other companies openly purchase and sell tissue such as dura matter and fascia lata.[38]

Furthermore, people get a tax deduction for donating money for research to find a cure for AIDS or cancer. Isn't this a public policy that "rewards" giving a gift? A gift aimed at maximizing life?

One objection holds that it is permissible to allow payment for renewable bodily tissue but not for nonrenewable tissue. The Bellagio Report skewers this objection nicely:

> The counter-argument that unlike solid organs, blood and sperm are self-renewing body parts is not telling, for if the risk to health in selling one kidney is truly minimal (which it is, at least in developed countries), then much of the relevance of the distinction disappears. By the same token, on what grounds may blood or bone be traded on the open market but not cadaveric kidneys?[39]

AGAINST FINANCIAL INCENTIVES: GOD'S WILL

The literature in transplant medicine and medical ethics reveals four major direct arguments against offering any kind of monetary incentives to increase organ transfers. Direct arguments claim that offering financial incentives to increase organ transfers is inherently wrong (indirect arguments don't claim it is inherently wrong, but that the cumulative consequences will be bad).

So what might make an act intrinsically wrong? The most general argument is that an act violates the command of God. This argument assumes that God exists, that His commands can be known, and that one of His commandments is a prohibition on buying and selling organs for transplantation.

Professor B. Teo, a Roman Catholic theologian, argued in 1992 that,

> the Catholic viewpoint also rejects all proposals to subject human body parts as objects of payment and as commodities of exchange. Allowing commerce in human body parts is not only disrespectful of human dignity but would also, in the words of Pope John-Paul II, "amount to the dispossession or plundering of a body" (*L'Osservatore Romano*, June 24, 1991). Furthermore, it would be corrosive of community. Communal bonds and relationships are built on compassion, goodwill, and altruism. Payment for body parts would undermine these values by transforming communal relationships into one of contractual buying and selling, thereby dissolving community.[40]

Professor Teo also says that selling organs allows the rich to exploit the poor (an objection that is muted with rewarded cadaveric donation or a regulated system between adults).

The main direct moral argument in Professor Teo's statement is that selling organs is "disrespectful of human dignity." (The others are indirect arguments, to be considered later.) So what is it about making a part of the body an object of commercial exchange that makes it "disrespectful of human dignity"? At the beginning of this article, Teo writes "Catholic tradition sees human life as a precious gift of God." The thrust of his article is that, if (1) life is a precious gift of God, then (2) the means to preserving it should not be bought or sold.

It is hard to see how (2) follows from (1). Just about everything in medicine can be construed to be a means of preserving life, and there are very few such services for which physicians are not reimbursed. Although the commercial aspect of such services is often concealed from patients by that form of prepaid, group medical coverage known as "medical insurance," that the service cannot be obtained without such fees being exchanged is well known to those without such coverage.

Moreover, if commercialization of organ procurement might increase the number of lives saved, how can increasing the number of lives saved be prohibited by appealing to the premise that life is a gift? Isn't some kind of primitive, religious fatalism lurking behind this objection, that is, that we either live or die at God's whim and that it is hubris for humans to try to do anything about it?

Of course, we should respect the value of life. If so, and if respecting God's will is against this value, are we supposed to believe that it is God's will for those waiting for a transplant to die rather than have families of brain-dead patients receive money? This conclusion seems to have God's will respecting dead bodies more than the lives of needy patients.

THE RIGHT KIND OF MOTIVE

Paying money to families to increase organ donation is considered immoral because it appeals to the wrong kind of motives in the people who consent. What is the right kind of motive? The answer, of course, is altruism. The official view in medicine, what I call *presumed altruism*, asserts that humans are altruistic and should give to one another unselfishly, especially when life itself is at stake. Clergy say that this is God's plan for helping mankind. Some philosophers and economists say that public policy must both assume some bit of altruism in humans and encourage it to flourish.

Presumed altruism is behind the position that the main reason why people don't donate is because of ignorance and, therefore, what we need is more education. In other words, people would donate if only they were educated enough about the need and lack of risks to themselves.

This position does not seem to be true. Over the past three decades, millions upon millions of dollars and thousands of persuasive pieces in the print and visual media have educated North Americans about the great need for organ donors, and indeed, large percentages of people in theory say they would donate. But when asked in actual cases, only a small percentage do.

So it seems that the present system is not working to meet demand. Put somewhat dramatically, no amount of pleading, of agonized chest-beating, of doleful pictures of dying children, seems likely to increase significantly the number of donated organs. Put more dramatically, we could ask what sane system allows thousands of good organs to go to the worms each year, when there are untried ways to increase organ donation?

In fact, the situation worsens each year. Over the past decade, there have been fewer brain-dead patients from head trauma (a primary source of organs) because of laws requiring airbags, mandatory use of seatbelts, helmets for motorcycle drivers, and safer construction of vehicles. Meanwhile, as medicine has kept more and more people alive, the number of patients needing transplants soars. For example, nearly four million Americans were infected with hepatitis C in 1999. These are people who might one day need a liver transplant.[41]

In philosophy, the kind of ethical theory assumed by presumed altruism champions impartiality, the idea that I should not be partial to my own family, kin, tribe, or nation, but treat all suffering beings the same and with equal moral worth. In theology, the kind of ethical theory champions *caritas*, or the virtues. Such theories, and the altruistic appeals based on them, have not worked well enough in organ donation, and if ethical theory is going to be anything other than an intellectual exercise, there must be some possibility of verification or falsification of it in real human life.

If sociobiologists such as E. O. Wilson are correct, human evolution has equipped humans with only a limited amount of altruism, generally extending only to the immediate circle of family, friends, and community (where *community* is defined by membership in a church, business, neighborhood, or profession). As the English philosopher G. J. Warnock writes about morality and the human predicament, "One may say for a start, mildly, that most human beings have some natural tendency to be more concerned about the satisfaction of their own wants . . . than those of others."[42] Not only does human nature have limited sympathy for others, Warnock asserts, but humans can also manifest complete indifference to the fate of others and active malevolence toward those seen in competition with themselves.

When these arguments are made, people always respond, "But education hasn't really been tried enough! It's too early to try financial incentives." To which it can be replied, "How much evidence is needed to falsify this claim? Can there *ever* be enough?"

Take donation of blood, for example. Altruistic donation of blood has actually *decreased* in the past decade, and we know that most hospitals and the American Red Cross have tried every conceivable educational tool to increase donation. It is important to note that the reasons for this decline do *not* concern increasing competition from vendors paying more for blood. Instead, with both parents of families working, with long commutes to distant suburban homes, and with employers increasingly unwilling to subsidize medicine by donating on-the-job time to allow donation of blood (and for many other reasons), U.S. donation of blood has dropped from 13.2 million pints in 1992 to 12.3 million in 1997, despite the large growth in population.[43] As the year 2000 approached, lack of regular donation of blood in the United States approached a crisis, causing creation of a special government panel to look into ways of making changes.[44]

In his review of Titmuss's book, economist Kenneth Arrow wrote that:

> like many economists, I do not want to rely too heavily on substituting ethics for self-interest. I think it best on the whole that the requirement of ethical behavior be confined to those circumstances where the price system breaks down. . . . Wholesale usage of ethical standards is apt to have undesirable consequences. We do not wish to use up recklessly the scarce resource of altruistic motivation.[45]

In retrospect, Arrow may have had the more accurate view about human nature. Altruistic behavior is in limited supply and should not be abused by being taken for granted.

Consider registering to be a bone marrow donor. To register is to imply and to accept a commitment to donate, should one match a needy recipient. To donate is potentially to save a life. On the other hand, donation requires a two-day hospital stay, puncture of one's hipbone by a long needle, loss of pay from work, and potential iatrogenic complications. Moreover, because it is so hard to find a good match, the donation will almost certainly help only a stranger, not anyone the donor knows. For these reasons and others, few people register, especially compared with the need for donors.

Bone marrow transplantation might increase if competent adults could be paid to be donors. Because there is only a one in sixty thousand chance of a match occurring between a random donor and a recipient, and because of the risks just mentioned, many people will never receive such transplants unless more donors can be encouraged to come forward. If payment causes only 1 percent of Americans to become donors, that might put two hundred fifty thousand donors in the market who are not there now, and that will be enough to create hundreds of good matches. The same point holds for kidney donation.

Does adding financial incentives to altruism always create a worse system? Consider pro bono medicine by physicians before Medicare began in 1965 ("Medicare" is federally funded for Americans over 65; "Medicaid" is run by each state for indigent patients and may be poorly funded.)

Medicine before Medicare is often misremembered with fond nostalgia by elderly physicians, who think patients had it better, in contrast to today, when "government bureaucrats run everything." The old system made physicians feel good, but the elderly poor were acutely dependent on the local physician, who might or might not be charitable. In truth, the elderly greatly feared sickness then, and they feared being dependent on the intermittent charity of whatever physician happened to be around until he retired, moved, or died. Hugely successful, Medicare removed such fears from old age.

Later, the Medicaid program compensated physicians for previously free, compassionate medical care of the poor. In these state-based systems, partially funded by the federal government, physicians no longer treat "charity" patients without compensation. (Ironically, it is largely the working poor between eighteen and sixty-five who don't have medical coverage and, hence, who aren't eligible for most organ transplants.)

In view of what has happened with Medicare and Medicaid, we can use the history to see that not every change in reimbursement in medicine away from pure altruism is insidious. Mixed systems can work well. If you look at the numbers of patients helped, anyone can see that the compensation of physicians for care of the elderly and poor was a great step in the right direction.

MORALLY WRONG IN ITSELF

Offering financial incentives is most often said to be wrong because it makes commodities of humans, their bodies, or parts of the human body. This claim is made over and over again in the literature by surgeons and others. But such surgeons generally do not articulate *why* it was wrong to allow selling kidneys, they merely repeatedly say that it is "obviously" wrong.

Consider the following summation of arguments against commercialization in one medical journal specializing in transplantation:

> [To permit payment for kidneys would be wrong because it would be] the commodification of the body; treating the body as an "it" rather than as a "self"; diminution of altruism in society at large; the coarsening of society's view of other persons; and so on. All these become a greater burden on society if human life is cheapened by putting a price on living human organs.[46]

This typical argument is more assertion than reason. Consider another, similar summation:

> To market organs for transplantation, or any other purpose, would be to market pieces of the self, pieces of the person, to put a price on human life and health best thought of as priceless. [Moreover] . . . neither transplantation itself, nor efficiency in the supply of organs, should be viewed as goods worth any price. There is a

widely shared perception, reflected in our laws and other public policies, that some things should not be allowed in the marketplace.[47]

Most of the above-mentioned statements assert that it is wrong to think of a part of the body as something that could be sold and that it would be better if people were altruistic. Of course, such arguments always leave out the people who are dying for lack of a transplant. Moreover, the last quotation appeals to a "perception" of the wrongness of commercialization, yet one 1992 poll found that most Americans favor some sort of financial incentive to increase organ donation, especially from cadavers.[48]

A variation of this argument holds that the human body is sacred and should not be "desecrated," that is, the human body is "the Temple of the Lord." Such a view implies that bodies should be left intact at death and not "violated" by surgeons. This view has a long history, originating at the beginnings of anatomy in opposing vivisection. At its heart, however, this argument is not materially different from the first argument that God is against commercial incentives for organs.

It is striking how often people in religion make reductionist assumptions, for example, as if the self is "nothing but" bodily states. (A similar assumption by religious leaders appears in chapter 7, where such people argue against a patent on human genes because it makes a commodity of "the sacred.")

It is true that Christians believe in resurrection of the body, but surely they don't believe that the body resurrected is the body actually buried. Few Christians believe that their resurrected body will be the one with the severed spinal cord or the emaciated shell of their one hundred five-year-old body. Instead, they believe that God restores the body in Heaven to its youthful prime. Given that God is omnipotent, he surely can also restore any organs then that were removed to benefit others on earth.

To give the argument its due, there is always some danger with commercial incentives that society's altruism will be diminished, that human beings will see each other in less respectful terms, and that human life will be "cheapened." It should be stressed that the important question here is not whether there is *any* danger, but whether the danger is so clear and great that we are willing to let thousands of people die to avoid it.[49] If we allow financial incentives for cadaveric donation, or even in a regulated system between adults, some people will be offended, some poor people will be exploited, some people will make bad decisions, and some surgeons will be unscrupulous. All that is true, but that harm must be balanced against first, eliminating the harms in our present system (deceit, harms to live donors, etc.) and second, saving the lives of many people.

Besides, over the past thirty years, every time a change occurs in medical ethics, critics have predicted such dangers, but they almost never come true.

Hence, the onus of proof would seem to be on those making the dire predictions.

WRONG KIND OF SYSTEM

Some critics of financial incentives, such as the religious critics mentioned above and philosopher Samuel Gorovitz of Syracuse University, argue that financial incentives would create the wrong kind of society in America and the wrong kind of world system. They want to avoid a world where desperate people are forced to sell their organs to get by. Rather than give in to such desperation, they believe that taking the moral high road is better, building caring and altruism into the system.[50] Gorovitz also said, "a public health policy that allows for situations in which individuals are motivated to sell an irreplaceable part of themselves to achieve their objectives is an unwise social policy. It is unwise largely because it fails to nurture a noncompetitive, compassionate, collective response to the plight of those in desperate circumstances."[51]

Gorovitz argued this way in testifying before Congressman Albert Gore's subcommittee in 1983 and was influential in getting a pure market system for organ donations banned. But his success may have had more to do with a "yuck" response to Barry Jacobs's proposed business than to the quality of his arguments. Four years later, Thomas Murray (who in 1999 replaced Daniel Callahan as head of the Hastings Institute) followed Titmuss's work and argued in an influential article that markets for organs destroy the moral and social dimensions of social life.[52]

There is some merit in these objections, especially as objections to a pure market in organs between competent adults who buy and sell organs. One way to look at these objections differently is to see them as issues across the planet, to which I now turn.

INTERNATIONAL INJUSTICE

It is always objected that allowing competent adults to sell their own kidneys would create international injustice, as poor people from undeveloped countries would sell their organs to the rich (this situation is claimed to have occurred in Italy and India).[53] Such very poor patients cannot give real consent, and even if they can, we should not encourage a world where conditions are so miserable that people must sell parts of their bodies to survive.

Bioethicist William May makes this point well by reminding us of the injustice that occurred during the American Civil War, when the rich were able to buy exemptions from service and commissions. Similarly, students from middle-class families could go to college to avoid the Vietnam War, while poor kids went off to die or be maimed.

This argument has a factual basis. A strong piece of evidence about how such a system could quickly develop into an organ-conduit from poor people in undeveloped countries to middle-class people in developed ones is how international blood banks operated in Managua, Nicaragua, in the mid-1970s.[54] In a remarkably short time, poor Nicaraguans were being systematically "bled" for the benefit of U.S. plasma companies, and it is easy to see how a similar process could develop for organs in today's global economy.

University of Pennsylvania bioethicist Arthur Caplan, a leading bioethicist whose work on organ transplants is highly respected within bioethics, also thinks it would be unfair to create an international system where people could sell a kidney or receive a donation for a deceased person's organs but never be a candidate themselves for such an organ transplant.[55]

I think he is right. Should there be an international market among competent adults, it would be unavoidable that North Americans and Europeans would be buying human organs from people in undeveloped countries. While we can enforce laws and regulations about brain death and organ donation in advanced countries, we cannot similarly control what happens in underdeveloped countries. On an international scale, a system with financial incentives might encourage abuses through murder of vulnerable people. The Chinese military has almost certainly killed prisoners for the simple reason they were a "match" for a rich person needing an organ transplant. In North America, we should refuse to accept organs from outside our country that were obtained as a result of financial incentives. Inside our boundaries, we should similarly bar organ transfers from anyone who is suspected of having been murdered or from anyone who committed suicide.

But what about a market that functions just in the United States between competent adults? At this time, it's probably not necessary because instituting a national system of rewarded cadaveric donation might solve the immediate problem of lack of supply. In a system allowing sales between competent adults, it would be hard to prevent problems, such as sales by recently arrived immigrants or mentally unstable people.

Before we choose a pure market, we should try a regulated market between competent adults. Although governments are not good at setting the price that will motivate people to sell or buy an organ, at least the U.S. or Canadian government could find a way to ensure that rich people do not have unfair advantages, that working people without insurance are eligible for transplants, and that sellers are competent to give informed consent. Although I'm not personally in favor of governments generally doing these things in medicine, in this case it could be acceptable should cadaveric donation fail to generate enough organs.

The real practical alternative I would like to push in the final pages of this chapter is rewarded cadaveric donation. This system has the fewest possible harms, the greatest advantages for waiting patients, and the greatest chance of actual implementation. As such, my remaining remarks focus on it.

REWARDED CADAVERIC DONATION AND INJUSTICE

Wouldn't the same problems of injustice arise about rewarded cadaveric donation? If we should ban financial incentives to increase transfers from poor adults to rich ones, why shouldn't we also ban such incentives to increase transfers from cadaveric donation? After all, rich and middle-class people almost always have good medical coverage and would be little influenced by payments under a thousand dollars.

Legally, paying relatives for cadaveric organs raises no special problems not already raised by relatives greedy for inheritances. As Gloria Banks concludes in her excellent legal review of commercialized organ transfers, "These concerns can be overcome by the enforcement of existing criminal statutes and the enactment of other appropriate punitive and regulatory measures to deter such conduct."[56] Some of these issues are problems of fine-tuning, not major obstacles.

Caplan argues that, "Before calling for markets or compensation for cadaver parts, the transplant community and organized medicine at least have an obligation to ensure that every American in need has an equal chance to receive a transplant."[57] For Caplan, the poor should not be able to receive money for agreeing to the transplant of a brain-dead patient's organs until they are able to receive such a transplant, regardless of their medical coverage, whether they work, or (presumably) whether their parents were U.S. citizens. (It should be noted than all Americans are eligible for kidney transplants, which are paid for by the federal government.)

This is an argument that can be countered. There is a frustrating tendency of egalitarians to pick on any new medical advance for their beliefs. But we always need to ask, not just of new reproductive advances, but of any new advance in medicine, why should it be made available equally to all? Whether it is a new drug for arthritis, Viagra, in vitro fertilization, or genetic enhancement, why should any new advance be delayed until it can be made equally available to all?

It would be one thing if we had a national single-payer medical system supported by a national tax to pay for it, but we don't. Different people pay for different levels of benefits, and therefore they are entitled to different levels of benefits. To deny this is like saying that car manufacturers shouldn't be able to sell Camrys until the government buys every poor person a car.

Caplan also argued in 1997 that offering financial incentives for cadaveric donation now would, in his opinion, "offend" people.[58] He rightly points out that offering such incentives contradicts "forty years of public policy . . . [during which] health professionals and the public have repeatedly been told that the 'gift of life' must be made solely on the basis of altruistic, voluntary choice."

But Caplan doesn't emphasize how unsuccessful such a policy has been or that we've never really tried financial incentives. And as said, it is much more difficult to prove that rewarded *cadaveric* donation will harm community morale and fellow-feeling, especially to such an extent that thousands of people should die to support such feelings. However, we should institute rewarded cadaveric donation only in North America, where we can properly ensure informed consent and lack of coercion.

Whether offering money for cadaveric donation is offensive also depends to a degree on who does the asking. Using sensitive, trained nurses has vastly increased rates of donation of corneas from brain-dead cadavers in Florida, where critics previously claimed that people wouldn't donate if asked directly (some states permit corneas to be taken without asking and without familial consent).[59] Financial incentives will have to be offered in a sensitive, respectful manner that does not erode trust and by professionals that families feel they can trust. Because this has been done in Florida with corneal donation, it can be done elsewhere for organ donation.

DISCOURAGEMENT OF ALTRUISM

Some critics fear that cash payments for organs could actually *decrease* available organs, as those who formerly would have donated altruistically become disenchanted. Relatives might think they have no right to personally profit from consenting to donation and hence, if they were offered money, would not consent.

This has not proven to be true with blood. Although almost everyone knows that he or she could theoretically sell his or her blood, the vast majority of blood in the United States comes from altruistic donation. There is no reason that two types of system cannot exist side by side, especially when both contribute to sustaining human life. People worried about profiting from consenting to cadaveric donation can specify that their money go to charity.

CONCLUSIONS

We could discuss other arguments against commercialism, mostly bad ones, such as the claim that urban legends will increase with commercialism. One such prevalent myth (which I hear every term from some student who swears it's true, because "a friend who wouldn't lie told me,") is that a college coed visits Atlanta and goes to a bar. The next day, she wakes up in pain in a motel room with a wound across her back because one of her kidneys has been cut out to be used for transplantation. Another such myth in Central America was once so popular that the State Department had to issue a warning to U.S. tourists: American surgeons, it was widely believed, were posing as tourists, kidnapping local babies, and shipping them to the United States to be organ sources.[60] It's not worthwhile discussing answers to such absurd beliefs. The appropriate response is not to make policy based on ignorance, but to get rid of false beliefs through education.

After all these considerations, I believe that a mixed commercial/altruistic system would be best for Americans. I also believe that offering financial incentives for cadaveric donation is ethically justified and practical. Instituting such a system would likely save thousands of American lives each year and cause little harm to living people.

At the very least, the government could offer one thousand dollars as a voucher, payable only to funeral homes for burial expenses. Such "in-kind" reimbursement systems may defuse the objection that "life" is being bought and sold or that it has a price tag.

Why not try this plan? Let's do empirical, not a priori, ethics and see if the experiment works. As mentioned, Pennsylvania plans to offer at least three hundred dollars for funeral expenses for cadaveric donations. Armchair critics, such as columnist Ellen Goodman, immediately cried that such payments were "cheapening life."[61] It's better, I guess, that hundreds of people die than to "cheapen life."

In 1997, the Bellagio Report studied this same issue. Like me, its commissioners were perplexed that the universal condemnations by transplant surgeons "failed to provide a rationale for their position." Although the reasons for their condemnation "appeared self-evident" to the surgeons, it did not seem so to the commissioners.

These commissioners were not convinced that rewarded giving would be the end of the world: "[We] found no unarguable ethical principle that would justify a ban on the sale of organs under all circumstances."[62] They concluded that a government-financed and government-regulated system of rewarded giving could work. As for the slippery slope, "a firm line can be maintained, between cadaveric and live donation, reducing the likelihood of moving down a slippery slope."

Here is my final idea: let's try a controlled experiment on a limited scale, say, in two states that are similar and with similar records of previous organ donation. In one state, we try rewarded cadaveric donation, funded by fees from automobile licenses and using skilled nurses and counselors to ask families to participate. In the other state, we do nothing new, and the state can serve as a true control. Why not try this test? What have we got to lose?

NOTES

1. "Payton in Waiting," *Birmingham News*, 17 February 1999, A13; "Payton Dies at 45," *New York Times*, 2 November 1999, A1.

2. Seth Hettena, "Teen Home after Three Quadruple Transplants," AP, *Birmingham News*, 18 December 1998, 5A.

3. Richard Batchelor, "Discussion on Organ Commerce," *Transplantation Proceedings* 22, no. 3 (June 1990): 935.

4. "Indian Kidney Trade," TED Case Studies, http://gurukul.ucc.american.edu/TED/

5. Richard A. Epstein, "Transplantation: The Supply Side," *Mortal Peril: Our Inalienable Right to Health Care?* (Reading, Mass.: Addison-Wesley, 1997), chapter 11, 255.

6. Although this is no longer done for livers, pancreases, and kidneys, for which we have twenty-four hours to transplant safely, it is still done for hearts.

7. D. J. Rothman et al., "The Bellagio Task Force Report on Transplantation, Bodily Integrity, and the International Traffic in Organs," *Transplantation Proceedings* 29 (1997): 2741.

8. Douglas Starr, *Blood: An Epic History* (New York: Knopf, 1998), chapter 11.

9. Ibid., 192–5.

10. Gloria J. Banks, "Legal and Ethical Safeguards: Protection of Society's Most Vulnerable Participants in a Commercialized Organ Transplantation System," *American Journal of Law and Medicine* (1995): 45–110.

11. Quoted from Samuel Gorovitz, "Testimony before the House Subcommittee on Investigation and Oversight," 9 November 1983, and reprinted in *Biomedical Ethics Reviews*, ed., James Humber and Robert Almeder (Clifton, N.J.: Humana Press, 1985), 7.

12. Starr, *Blood*, 228.

13. Ibid., chapter 13.

14. Of course, it is possible that an unknown agent is being transmitted now in blood, as in the early days of HIV infection and, hence, that blood donors still need to have good motives. I owe this point to Chuck Patrick of the Alabama Organ Center.

15. Council of Transplantation Society, *Lancet* 2, no. 715, 1985.

16. Rothman et al., "Bellagio Report," 2739.

17. This statistic is from the web site of the United Network for Organ Sharing (UNOS) in 1984.

18. C. R. Eisendrath, "Used Body Parts: Buy, Sell, or Swap?" *Transplantation Proceedings* 24, no. 5 (24 October 1992): 2212–4.

19. Actually, the raw numbers from UNOS say almost five thousand Americans die while waiting for transplants, but because hearts and lungs can be transferred from cadavers and because not all kidney and liver patients could be matched even if the organs were available, I have used the very conservative number of three thousand American deaths per year, or forty thousand since 1988.

20. Kant, of course, might not agree. But I also think that rewarded cadaveric donation is a maxim that reasonable people could adopt as a universal maxim, for reasons to be sketched out in the rest of this chapter.

21. Judith Jarvis Thomson, "The Trolley Problem," *Rights, Retribution and Risks: Essays in Moral Theory,* ed. W. Parent (Cambridge, Mass.: Harvard University Press, 1986).

22. "Bargain Kidneys," *New Scientist,* no. 2188 (29 May 1999): 5, referring to a study by Eugene Schweitzer at the University of Maryland Medical Center in Baltimore. This assumes a transplanted kidney lasts more than three years, a reasonable assumption.

23. Peter Singer, "Altruism and Commerce," *Philosophy and Public Affairs* 2, no. 3 (Winter 1973): 313.

24. Lloyd Cohen, *Increasing the Supply of Transplant Organs* (New York: R. G. Landes, 1995), 92.

25. Epstein, *Mortal Peril,* 260.

26. See Institute of Medicine, *Non-Heart-Beating Organ Transplantation: Medical and Ethical Issues in Procurement* (Washington, D.C.: National Academy Press, 1997); also, the *Kennedy Institute of Ethics* 3, no. 2; the University of Wisconsin Medical Center has been procuring organs for years using this protocol, according to a *60 Minutes* story in April 1997. On the issues of changing definitions of brain death for adults and anencephalics, see Gregory Pence, chapters 1 and 14, *Classic Cases in Medical Ethics: Accounts of the Cases that Shaped Medical Ethics,* third edition (New York: McGraw-Hill, 2000).

27. Christiaan Barnard, quoted by Peter Hawthorne, *The Transplanted Heart* (Johannesburg, South Africa: Keartland Publishers, 1968), 84–5.

28. When Jack Burcham, the fourth recipient of a Jarvik-7™ artificial heart entered the operating room, surgeon William DeVries discovered that the device wouldn't fit inside Burcham's chest. When the patient left the OR, "his chest, draped with sterile dressing, . . [was] only partly closed around the device." Gideon Gill, "Burcham Dies after Blood Accumulates in Chest," *Louisville Courier-Journal,* 26 April 1985. For more, see Pence, "Artificial Hearts," *Classic Cases,* chapter 12.

29. Cohen, *Increasing the Supply,* 5. This passage discusses the "opting out" problem. This country presently also has the "opting in" problem, i.e., it is difficult to make one's wishes about organ transplantation or cadaveric donation known nationally, especially given that people over their lifetimes move from state to state, or even country to country.

30. A. Bass, "New Liver Transplants; Pressure on Parents," *Boston Globe,* 17 December 1989, 1, 75; quoted in Rene Fox and Judith Swazey, *Spare Parts: Organ Replacement in American Society* (Oxford: Oxford University Press, 1992), 52.

31. David Plank, "Nana Gives Gift of Life," *Newsday,* 29 July 1993, 6.

32. M. R. Tonelli, "Ethical Considerations in the Treatment of Cystic Fibrosis," *Current Opinions in Pulmonary Medicine,* 3, no. 6 (November 1997): 420–4.

33. V. Fourbister, "Living Donors Dramatize Risk vs. Need," *American Medical News,* 20 September 1999, 1.

34. The death was confirmed by Dr. Jean Edmond in Fourbister, "Living Donors."

35. Denise Grady, "The New Organ Donors Are Living Strangers," *New York Times*, 20 September 1999, A1.

36. Ibid.

37. Rothman et al., "Bellagio Report," 2741.

38. Ibid.

39. Ibid.

40. B. Teo "Organ Donation and Transplantation: A Christian Viewpoint," *Transplantation Proceedings* 24, no. 5 (October 1992): 2114.

41. John Gerome, "Hepatitis C Rise Triggers Search for New Treatments," *Birmingham News*, 27 September 1999, 1D.

42. G. J. Warnock, *The Object of Morality* (London: Methuen, 1971), 21.

43. Avram Goldstein, "Blood Supply Declines; Alarm Raised," *Washington Post*, Internet site, 7 June 1999.

44. Eric Nagourney, "Blood Shortage: Answer Scarce, Too," *New York Times*, 5 October 1999, D8.

45. Quoted from Singer, "Altruism and Commerce," 318.

46. J. B. Dossetor, "Rewarded Gifting: Is It Ever Ethically Acceptable?" *Transplantation Proceedings* 24, no. 5, (October 1992): 2094.

47. E. W. Keyserlingk, "Human Dignity and Donor Altruism: Are They Compatible with Efficiency in Cadaveric Human Organ Procurement?" *Transplantation Proceedings* 22, no. 3, (June 1990): 1005.

48. A. Guttmann and R. D. Guttmann, "Sale of Kidneys for Transplantation: Attitudes of the Health-Care Profession and Public," *Transplantation Proceedings* 24, no. 5 (October 1992): 2108.

49. I owe this way of making this point to James Rachels.

50. Samuel Gorovitz, "Global Objections to Kidney Sales: A Response to Professor Humber," *Biomedical Ethics Reviews*, eds. James Humber and Robert Almeder (Clifton, N.J.: Humana Press, 1985), 33.

51. Gorovitz, "Global Objections," 32.

52. Thomas Murray, "Gifts of the Body and Needs of Strangers," *Hastings Center Report*, 17 (1987): 35.

53. M. Eilli et al., "Developing Countries as the Major Future Source of Living Donor Renal Transplants," *Transplantation Proceedings* 24, no. 5 (October 1992): 2110.

54. Starr, *Blood*, 231ff.

55. Arthur Caplan, "No Sale: Markets, Organs, and Tissues," *Am I My Brother's Keeper? The Ethical Frontiers of Biomedicine* (Bloomington: Indiana University Press, 1997), 97–100.

56. Gloria J. Banks, "Legal and Ethical Safeguards: Protection of Society's Most Vulnerable Participants in a Commercialized Organ Transplantation System," *American Journal of Law and Medicine* 21, no. 1 (1995): 77.

57. Caplan, "No Sale," 98.

58. Ibid., 97.

59. Personal communication to author from Jason Woody, executive director/CEO, Central Florida Lions Eye and Tissue Bank, 12 December 1997. One of the largest corneal banks in the world, this bank shipped nine thousand corneas overseas in 1996 and obtained consent from all families for taking corneas.

60. For more, see the many books falsifying urban legends by University of Utah professor Jan Brunvald. See also Benjamin Radford, "Bitter Harvest: The Organ Snatching Urban Legends," *Skeptical Inquirer* 23, no. 3 (May/June 1999): 34–9.

61. Ellen Goodman, "No Money for Transplants," *Birmingham News*, 9 June 1999, A9.

62. Rothman et al., "Bellagio Report," 2741.

4

RE-CREATING MOTHERHOOD: BUYING REPRODUCTIVE HELP

"My husband told me, 'This is something you can do,' and I knew at that moment that he was right."

—"Mary" (on working as a paid, surrogate mother) in Helena Ragone, *Surrogate Motherhood: Conception in the Heart*

The folly of taboos long banished is easy to see. Now that other people have done the hard work of eradicating them, they are easy to mock. Challenging and changing them in your own time is another matter.

One of our current taboos concerns the merits of paid reproductive help. Almost all the publicity and discussion of this activity imply that it is bad. Our foremost bioethicists, physicians, and politicians imply that paid reproductive help is always unsavory and, at worst, destructive to children.

As I will argue throughout this book, I believe that such simplistic attitudes should be challenged. They almost never advance human progress. If we go back to an earlier time, we can appreciate the damage done by such simplistic moralism.

In 1864 physician J. Marion Sims sat out the Civil War by practicing in London and serialized his views on gynecology in England's best medical journal, the *Lancet*. In it, Sims debated Spencer Wells, England's leading physician, on the wisdom of obtaining a full view of the operating site in a vaginal operation. While Dr. Wells admitted the wisdom of this approach for the pharyngeal tract (women didn't mind surgeons looking down their throats, he averred), he claimed that a "modest woman" much preferred if the vaginal operation "can be done under the bedclothes, without any exposure." Sims, who decades before had invented the speculum to assist in performing such surgery, was accustomed to defending himself against charges of indecency. "The use of the speculum," he had replied, "is delicate or indelicate only according to the manner of him who uses it."[1]

Sims is a controversial figure in medicine. Some historians consider him a racist. He perfected therapeutic surgeries on women for whom birth had torn the tissue between the rectum and uterus, leaving them with constant infections. This condition caused great distress and discomfort in these women, rendering them unable to function in normal life. Although he tried to cure this condition on both white and black women, his repeated surgeries were ultimately only successful with black female slaves. His sutures healed the vesico-vaginal fistula, allowing these women to return to normal life. He can be faulted for having different standards for white women and black slave women and for believing that the black slave women were tougher by nature than the white women they served.

When he published his major medical book, *Clinical Notes on Uterine Surgery*, physicians condemned it for its frank, natural, clinical language.[2] The book described the best positions for examining female patients, as well as instruments Sims had created for operating on gynecological disease. The book's really controversial sections discussed ideas for curing infertility.

Sims refused to discuss infertility and sexual relations in Latin, as was customary among the physicians of his day, preferring the use of plain English in order to educate couples. He shocked his colleagues by adopting experimental methods, such as having infertile couples engage in intercourse in the next room, then examining the wife afterward for presence of mucus and sperm.[3] As a result of these examinations, Sims was one of the only physicians of his day to claim that a potent man could be infertile (today we believe that men and women contribute equally to the occurrence of infertility).

As Sims often experienced firsthand, moral censure can be a weapon against medical progress. Especially in reaction to advances in human reproduction, moral criticism can wound both the villain and the hero. "Did it ever occur to you," Sims asked in his presidential address to the annual meeting of the American Medical Association in 1876, "that [our Code of Ethics] is capable of being used as an engine of torture and oppression?"[4]

Fortunately, Sims had another criterion of success. Despite denouncements of his work from pulpits and from jealous medical rivals, women everywhere flocked to him. When he visited Europe, countesses and duchesses were his patients; the empress of France sought him out. Whether practicing in France,

England, or the United States, Sims was besieged by women of means begging to be his patients.

A new appreciation of Sims has recently begun, in contrast to the usual simplistic portrayal of him by historians of medicine. One example of this appreciation is a fine new history of infertility by two sisters, one a historian and the other a medical professor of obstetrics and gynecology. They write,

> In spite of the opposition of his colleagues in the 1860s to his single-minded emphasis on surgery, however, within a decade or so his views would come to prevail. One reason is that his ideas seemed to "work," perhaps not in the sense that he made the sterile fertile (although enough of his patients conceived to enable him to develop a reputation for success), but that he convinced his patients that his instruments and his surgical expertise provided them with more hope of relief— from their pelvic pain, their dysmenorrhea, and their sterility—than any dietary prescriptions, gradual instrumental therapy, or self-help could do. The fact that he actually had been the first to cure vesico-vaginal fistula, an accomplishment of genuine significance that had released many afflicted women from a lifetime of suffering, gave credence to his well-substantiated claims. With the Woman's Hospital as an institutional base . . . Sims had created a small corps of "women's surgeons" who became identified with the cure of women's reproductive disorders.[5]

Eventually, Sims died honored and famous, although his rivals attempted to defame him even after his death.

The previous chapter argued that nothing is wrong with paying families to save lives by transplanting the living human tissue of deceased persons. Similarly, this chapter shall argue that nothing is wrong with paying for sperm, eggs, or gestational help to create human lives.

Amazingly, many physicians and bioethicists believe that (despite the successes) the influence of money has been a bad thing in assisted reproduction; they think that because creation of life has moved from pure altruism to altruism-plus-compensation, reproductive medicine has become tainted, unnatural, and wrong. The same kind of thinking predicts that if organ donation moves from pure altruism to altruism-plus-compensation, bad things will occur. Yet the truth is just the opposite: private fees for reproductive services have been the catalyst for almost all breakthroughs in reproductive medicine.

THE MEDIA AND REPRODUCTIVE ETHICS

Innovations in reproductive ethics are normally brought to our attention in sensationalistic ways. The way this is done today is little different than it was a hundred years ago.

"Internet Offers Embryos by Mail!!" So screamed the May 10, 1998, head-line in Melbourne, Australia's Sunday *Herald Sun*.[6] (Note: All of the quotes in this section come from this article.) Such headlines attract attention and imply that something truly awful is at hand. In this story, it helped that older Aus-tralians for some years had been feeling that they had fallen behind in the com-puter revolution and that the Internet-via-computers was the purveyor of this evil. It also helped that the site of evil was the United States, which the Aus-tralian media loved to criticize for its excesses of commercialism. The coup de grâce was that the embryo was available for a fee of four thousand dollars.

For traditional Australians, bewildered by a changing world and used to a na-tional medical system that provides all medical services for free (even in vitro fertilization), the reductio ad absurdum was right there: embryos created through in vitro fertilization without sex, an Internet where people talked to each other without ever meeting, "tiny babies" (embryos) available by air mail from the United States, and finally, human life reduced to a price. Other crit-ics on television called this "mail-order children, created to specifications."

Given the way this story was presented to them, so-called church and family groups in Australia reacted predictably—angrily, as if their world were being threatened. Getting their facts mixed up, they said that creating babies "by air mail" was abhorrent and that offering embryos for a fee this way was a "heart-less cash grab that disrespected the dignity of human life and children's welfare."

Actually, sperm still needed to meet egg to produce human embryos, and whether payment of money itself made the service "a heartless cash grab" cer-tainly begged a lot of questions.

What was true in the story was that some clinics offered web sites with pic-tures and profiles of past and prospective young females who were willing to undergo egg recovery and transfer for a fee. For an additional fee, a couple in another country could mail in the man's sperm, have it mixed with an egg of the selected woman, have an embryo created, have the embryo frozen, and have the embryo sent back to them via an overnight delivery service.

Of course, the story left out a lot. Creating and delivering an embryo is a far cry from having a live human baby. Most (80 percent per cycle) embryos used in assisted reproduction (AR) fail to implant or gestate in the uterus, so the hard part was still ahead. And, of course, embryos grow neither on trees nor in vats, so healthy females must be willing to gestate the embryos for nine months. Next, even if a healthy child results, it will not be a "mail-order child, created to specifications," because our knowledge of the way in which various genes-with-the-environment create a specific trait is mostly guesswork.

The writer of the *Herald Sun* story was horrified that infertile couples could choose the kind of embryo they wanted. But is there any other way? Why would we use a different standard than we have used for decades with adoption? Imagine that a Caucasian, American couple had no choice but to take the first embryo available. So they would end up with an embryo from whom? An Indonesian Muslim couple? Would that be the best option? Should public policy in assisted reproduction have as its major goal creating babies of mixed ethnicity and forcing such babies on unwilling couples? Neither the donating couple nor the receiving couple would likely be happy with those results.

The Australian paper was horrified that fees were paid to the staff of the fertility clinic and to the female source of the egg. Upon reflection, this is not such a hair-raising practice. Indeed, it seems to be the customary arrangement, because most people don't work for free. Yellow journalists and indignant academics may horrify their readers with information that women are being paid for such services—as if doing so were obviously demeaning—while omitting the equally obvious point that they think it's not wrong to be paid to write newspapers or to teach in college.

Finally, what was left out, and what reduces it from a the-sky-is-falling story to a variation-on-a-theme story, was the fact that the chances of this procedure actually producing a baby were so small. As mentioned, in vitro fertilization is not a very efficient procedure, and its success rate with thawed human embryos is even lower. In addition, only 10 percent of frozen sperm work with such a procedure (more on this later). Moreover, even fewer states require insurance companies to cover this procedure than did ten years ago, so it's mainly a cash-and carry (!) service, which most couples cannot afford. Despite the implications of the *Herald Sun* story, we are a long, long way from the time when the average couple can create a baby by looking up its future characteristics in some biological *J. Crew Catalog*.

In this case, one of the harshest critics was the Catholic Church in Australia, whose spokesman, Christopher Prowse, thundered,

> We see this as the commercialization of human life that insults the dignity of human life, which is a gift from God. You can't look at the issue of childless couples just from the couples' point of view. Children have rights, too, but they are never spoken about. Human embryos are the tiniest and most vulnerable of human life but they are becoming fair game for a lot of people seeking to profit from this unethical industry.[7]

And so the criticism goes that human embryos have status, in fact have interests that trump those of childless couples. And the solution? An ally of the Church, one Helen Woods of the Australian Family Association, suggested that if fewer women had abortions and if adoption was made easier, the whole problem would be solved. Moreover, Woods continued, regarding the welfare of the children created from such embryos, "How do you explain to the child that it [*sic*] was formed through mail order?"

This seems very shortsighted, as if it's better not to exist than to have had the semen and egg that created you travel around the world. As if no natural combination of egg and sperm ever came together in the backseat of a '54 Chevy by accident. Woods offers simplistic solutions (don't abort; adopt more), while she imagines the perceived trauma of having been sent through the mail as an embryo (Hmmm!! I wonder if I could sue my mother for the "trauma" I experienced as an embryo while traveling down her fallopian tube?).

The sad fact is that we haven't progressed much from the sensationalist days of William Randolph Hearst. Visual and print media still present new reproductive options in breathless, sky-is-falling language, scaring people and making them think that the family is constantly under attack. Personally, I believe that new forms of assisted reproduction are just new ways of creating families and, for the vast majority of couples, creating traditional families.

GOOD OF THE CHILD

Of course, there is some truth in the criticisms of the Catholic Church when its spokesperson says, "You can't look at the issue of childless couples just from the couples' point of view. Children have rights, too." Indeed, too much of the criticisms of new forms of assisted reproduction and their commercial versions focus on what it does or does not do for the parents and whether it's good or bad for those offering assistance. Rarely does its discussion focus on the good of the child.

However, we must tread carefully here, because "good of the child" is a loaded, ambiguous phrase. The usual assumption made by conservative critics of assisted reproduction is that the ideal way to be born is to be a child of married, heterosexual parents who carefully plan the pregnancy. Any deviation from this idea, for example, by introducing a third party (sperm or egg donor, surrogate), is held to be harmful to the resulting child.

Defenders of assisted reproduction point out that without innovative forms of assisted reproduction or paid assistants, the child would never have been born. Having life is better than having none, they retort. A child can't be "harmed" by being brought into existence. Sometimes such defenders retreat by asserting that as long as the adult doesn't later want to kill himself, or the baby's life is not one of total pain ("wrongful life"), it's better off existing than not.

Both views of child harming are problematic. According to the first, many children born on the planet are "harmed" by the process of conception, because their creation isn't planned or their parents aren't married. No doubt, conception as a result of planned sexual intercourse is a very good way to produce a baby, perhaps ideal. But, if this is considered the only moral way to produce a child, it might be good to remember that *many unplanned conceptions by ordinary people are immoral, far more than we might think* (indeed, even in seventeenth-century England, a third of all women were already pregnant when they got married).[8] On the other hand, the second view implies that a child can be very less-than-normal (e.g., suffer from fetal-maternal alcohol syndrome) and not be harmed, because otherwise he wouldn't have existed. This also seems far-fetched, especially if the parents or society could have exercised precautions that would have prevented the abnormality.

I believe the solution is to define *harm* neither as a departure from the ideal nor as equivalent to the worst-case outcome but as a departure from the *average*. A child born as a result of assisted reproduction should be seen as harmed if the child is less healthy than the average child born as a result of traditional coitus (estimating that about 1 percent of such traditionally conceived children have some kind of defect).

Based on this commonsensical definition of harm, I do not believe that most children conceived from anonymous sperm donors or egg transfers or children carried by surrogates are harmed by the fact that their origins differed slightly from those of other people. So even if the "best interests of the child" is the important moral standard by which to evaluate new forms of assisted reproduction, most new forms of AR turn out to be morally permissible.

HISTORICAL DIGRESSION
ABOUT FALSE IDEALS OF THE FAMILY

Many criticisms of the new forms of assisted reproduction or of paying for reproductive assistance assume that the ideal nuclear family is the one pictured in old television comedies, such as *Leave It to Beaver* or *The Donna Reed Show*. Although students know that such perfect families rarely exist today, most falsely believe that something like these nuclear families actually did exist in the past. They think that only recently did the nuclear family decline, because of working mothers, high rates of divorce, feminism, or lack of religious schooling. In her well-received surveys of U.S. family life over the past centuries, historian Stephanie Coontz contradicts these widespread beliefs. In *The Way We Never Were*, she writes,

> the middle-class Victorian family depended for its existence on the multiplication of other families who were too poor and powerless to retreat into their own little

oases and who therefore had to provision the oases of others. . . . For every nine-teenth-century middle-class family that protected its wife and child within the fam-ily circle, then, there was an Irish or a German girl scrubbing the floors in that mid-dle-class home, a Welsh boy mining coal to keep the home-baked goodies warm, a black girl doing the family laundry, a black mother and child picking cotton to be made into clothes for the family, and a Jewish or an Italian daughter in a sweatshop making "ladies" dresses or artificial flowers for the family to purchase.[9]

So the family pictured on *Leave It to Beaver* did not exist for most Americans at most times in history. It is also important to stress that we have little real ev-idence about the forms of child raising that work best. Again, I quote Coontz:

> There are limits to what parents can do to counter the effects of class position, eco-nomic pressures, working conditions, and the all-pervasive television. But the fact that parental power is limited makes parenting easier in some ways, too. As it turns out, time and individual initiative heal many of the wounds of childhood. A W. T. Grant Foundation study of aging found that many early life experiences, even seemingly devastating problems in childhood, had virtually no influence on well-being at age sixty-five. I am not saying that we should disregard the impact of our actions on our children, putting blind faith in time, luck, class advantages, or a child's natural resiliency. There are measurably different consequences of various parental behaviors and family patterns. But in many cases, researchers simply do not know what they're measuring or what significance the differences they are finding will have. Psychologist Lois Hoffman points out that "traits that seem mal-adaptive at one age may develop into strengths as the child matures, or the con-verse pattern may emerge."[10]

Coontz relates a study where researchers tracked kids to adolescence and pre-dicted which kids would be happy and which would be unhappy, based on their childhoods and the parenting they received.[11] The researchers *were wrong two-thirds of the time*, worse than if they had guessed randomly. They vastly overestimated the trauma resulting from the typical stresses of childhood, while they underestimated the lack of maturity that resulted from having a protected, stress-free adolescence.

It is very taboo today to acknowledge any evidence countering the prevailing wisdom about child development. In 1999, "family-values" conservatives attacked psychological studies showing that sexual abuse of adolescents and children is not universally damaging and that some victims of such abuse emerge as unscathed adults.[12] Similar studies in 1999 showed that most children do fine in homes with-out live-in fathers. Rather than seeing this as good news about the resilience of children or the effectiveness of therapy, conservatives attacked the messengers, vowing to revoke any federal funding of such studies by psychologists.

The point is that solid, empirical research is very scanty about what forms of child raising harm children. Many erroneous beliefs about child raising, both in the past and in the present, could stem from the pervasive influence of a few television shows.

These points are important to keep in mind when conservatives claim that children are harmed by new forms of child creation. Being raised on a kibbutz, in day care, or being gestated by a surrogate, might not be generally harmful at all. Speculation about the harm teenagers will suffer upon discovering that their conception or gestation differed slightly from traditional conceptions is just that, speculation.

PARADOX! SUCCESS FROM BANNING THE FUNDING OF RESEARCH ON EMBRYOS

More than twenty years ago, on July 28, 1978, a baby named Louise Brown was born to John and Lesley Brown in northern England, becoming the first baby born to have been outside the womb for a few hours as an embryo. This embryo was created in a petri dish from John's sperm and Lesley's egg.

Development of in vitro ("in glass") fertilization not only allowed previously infertile couples to have children but also allowed the study of live human embryos.[13] In vitro fertilization is inefficient (only about twenty of one hundred using it are able to create a baby with their own eggs and sperm), and earlier, worse results in the 1980s spurred research on embryos to increase rates of success.

In 1979, the obstetricians Howard and Georgeanna Jones established the first American in vitro fertilization (IVF) clinic at Eastern Virginia Medical School (EVMS). The then-sixtyish couple had been asked to leave Johns Hopkins because of Johns Hopkins' mandatory-retirement age, but when they went to EVMS, this "over-the-hill" couple founded the United States' most successful IVF clinic, producing a thousand successes over the next two decades. In October 1979, opponents of IVF jammed the auditorium of the Norfolk Public Health Department for a debate on the proposed program at EVMS, charging that it would inevitably lead to the destruction of "tiny human beings" and the "murder of tiny babies." The protesters envisioned mass production of artificially designed humans.

EVMS is a private institution, not subject to federal regulations, and so its program went forward, with the result that Elizabeth Carr was born (she is now a healthy nineteen-year-old in Westminister, Massachusetts). But the protests spooked some members of Congress, because this brouhaha piggybacked on a very different controversy.

In 1973, only months after the January *Roe v. Wade* decision, researchers used eight human fetuses obtained by hysterotomy in an attempt to develop an artificial placenta. The human fetuses weighed between 300 and 1,000 grams, and when the largest of them was placed in a warm saline solution, mimicking the amniotic fluid, it was described by the researchers as making frantic "gasping" efforts and limb-stretching movements as it died.[14] Another experiment studied the effects of lack of glucose on the fetal brain, a condition arising when a diabetic pregnant woman goes into shock. The heads of twelve nonviable fetuses were severed after the fetal heart had stopped but before anoxia had damaged the brain. These brains were successfully maintained, using artificial replacements for glucose.[15] These gruesome experiments were described for the nation by journalist Maggie Scarf in a Sunday magazine story in the *New York Times*.

The fundamentalist Protestant theologian Paul Ramsey called such experimentation "unconsented-to research on unborn babies" and condemned it in the most vehement way as a "tragical case of [research on] a dying" baby.[16] Given the sensationalistic way these experiments were reported, and given how closely they followed the legalization of abortion, it was predictable that antiabortion forces would strongly condemn them.

As a result of revelation of these experiments in 1974, Congress banned all federally funded research involving fetuses. Not knowing exactly when a mere embryo becomes a fetus, Congress banned experiments not only on late-term fetuses but also on embryos only a few minutes old. Since most experimentation in the United States was then federally funded, this ban was designed to stop U.S. research on assisted reproduction. Indeed, the ban continues in 1999.

England and Australia originally took a more liberal view, allowing public funding for research on human embryos up to fourteen days old. As a result, in the early 1980s Australian infertility companies led the world and began to license their expertise in franchises all over the world. But then the forces of repression set in, especially in Australia, where a national medical system was vulnerable to pressures from social conservatives over research on embryos. Also, and very important, because the Australian government paid for the infertility treatments of infertile couples, there was little private funding to subsidize IVF research.

In 1999, the debate about the status of embryos acquired new urgency when researchers made the stunning discovery of how to derive human stem cells from early human embryos. It is hard to exaggerate the benefits that might develop from embryo-derived stem cells. Stem cells are cells that develop very early in human embryos that can develop into any of hundreds of specialized cells required by the adult body. Doctors might be able to take a cell from the body of a person afflicted with Parkinson's disease or Alzheimer's disease and, through somatic cell nuclear transfer (a.k.a. cloning), replace the nucleus in a human egg. That is, scientists would create an embryo-clone of the patient and direct the resulting stem cells into becoming whatever kind of specialized cells the patient needed. Such cells would be a perfect match and would not be rejected by the patient's immune system. Such "therapeutic cloning" was recently endorsed by a British panel of scientists.[17]

Many clinics have hundreds, even thousands of human embryos stored in liquid nitrogen. If these embryos could be used for research that prevented even one kid from having cystic fibrosis or Tay-Sachs disease, wouldn't it be worth it? A fourteen-day-old embryo the size of the period at the end of a sentence is a far cry from an eight-month-old human fetus. Why is it morally valuable to protect hundreds of such nonfeeling human embryos? Why, if the cost of this protection is one, or twenty, children born with Down's syndrome, cystic fibrosis, or degenerative neurological diseases? Isn't such embryo worship idolatry? Because embryos don't perceive anything or feel pain, isn't their value purely rhetorical and symbolic?

OVERTURNING THE BAN?

Over the years, practical-minded scientists and advocates for the infertile have tried to get the U.S. ban overturned. During the mid-1970s, Congress avoided facing the controversial issues of research on human embryos by delegating approval to a noncongressional committee, the Ethics Advisory Board (EAB), which was charged with approving any such research paid for with federal funds.

The EAB concluded that some such research was morally permissible, but before its conclusions could be enacted, Ronald Reagan took office in 1980. Believing that the destruction of embryos could be likened to the destruction of fetuses in abortion, the Reagan and Bush administrations did not renew the EAB's charter, which ended in 1981. Hence, no human embryo research could be approved.

So did U.S. research into infertility stop? Obviously not. Everyone has read about the many breakthroughs that have occurred in U.S. infertility clinics— from creating babies from thawed embryos to sixty-three-year-old Aleci Keh successfully gestating a baby created from her husband's sperm and a young woman's egg. How did this happen?

With a ban on federal funding, if assisted reproduction was going to flourish in the United States, research would have to take place in private clinics that accepted no federal funds. Furthermore, since few states required insurance companies to pay for AR services, clinics would have to subsidize their research from fees paid by private clients.

At one time, many people doubted that couples would actually pay for AR services, especially if a couple's chances of achieving a baby were low. The past two decades have proved such skeptics spectacularly wrong. (Would we have the same results if we were to offer money for cadaveric organ donation? Maybe. It's worth a try!)

Such errors in understanding human nature show the colossal stupidity of trying to block the fulfillment of basic human desires. A priori, it might seem reasonable to ban AR services as "too expensive" or as "frivolous," because more pressing medical needs were unmet. If AR were regulated by bureaucrats or committees, such a judgment might easily have been made, because many people in the early 1980s considered IVF unnatural and an improper goal of medicine (indeed, many forms of AR are banned in Europe).

Fortunately, the freedom to spend one's money as one chooses to buy reproductive help was still available (it would later be curtailed after the Baby M surrogacy case). As a result, some couples decided to drive fifteen-year-old cars, rent apartments rather than buy houses, and go without vacations— all to be able to afford an attempt to conceive a child through AR. Now, perhaps a million U.S. couples *every year* pay for some form of assistance in AR clinics.

Ironically, and wholly without intent, *the ban on federal funding of AR research on human embryos jump-started rapid, creative innovation in AR.* This miscalculation by antireproductive choice forces created one of the fastest growing areas of U.S. medicine and resulted in stupendous breakthroughs, fueled in part by competition among AR clinics for success in creating babies.

An unintended but foreseeable by-product of the ban on federal funding for research on human embryos (with the resulting reliance of such clinics on funds generated by their paying patients) was that research in such clinics was not regulated by the NIH or reviewed by the ethics committee (the Institutional Review Board [IRB]), which the NIH required of institutions receiving federal funds.

So, should the ban be lifted? Although it would seem that I would be in favor of doing so, we should tread carefully here. The great danger is that if we were suddenly to allow federal funding of research on embryos up to fourteen days old, the change might come at the price of governmental regulation of all use of embryos in public *and private* clinics. That would be an exorbitant price to pay and would almost certainly produce worse results. At present with AR research in private clinics, we have unintentionally backed into a good arrangement where private infertility clinics finance their own research. Let us hope this arrangement continues without government interference.

BUYING SPERM: FROM MORAL CONTROVERSY TO BANALITY

One of the mantras of our time is "medical technology is changing faster than our ability to understand it." Today, people think that medicine is confronted by new moral issues that are unique to our time, when in truth, moral controversy over innovations in medicine has been relatively constant over the past 150 years.

Consider the history of insemination by donor sperm (AID). Around 1850, J. Marion Sims, while practicing in Montgomery, Alabama, artificially inseminated fifty-five Southern women with sperm from their husbands, in an attempt to help them have children.[18] He produced one pregnancy (but it later miscarried). He was forced to stop because of strident condemnation by physicians and clergy in his time. Later, when he detailed methods of AID in his textbook, the zealots in medicine grew white-hot with rage (some of them, in truth, worried about the shaky image of their profession at the time). Hence, the practice of artificial insemination was not adopted at that time.[19]

The net result? Hundreds, maybe thousands, of couples in the United States and Europe remained infertile, blaming each other for being barren, going childless not by choice but by fate, and not having heirs. Thousands of kids who might have been born, who today might have had hundreds of thousands of descendants, were not created.

It was not lack of medical knowledge or inadequate medical technology that blocked creation of these children. What blocked their creation were the anti-life morals that were pushed on society in the name of "the sacredness of life," of the "naturalness" of family creation, of our "way of life," of "God's will," and other glosses on the view that any variation from fatalistically determined conception leads to disaster.

In the 1890s, Brooklyn physician Robert Latou Dickinson was vilified for practicing AID. He persevered but was still accused of aiding and abetting "technological adultery." (Dickinson was also an early pioneer of contraception.) Earlier, in 1884, Dr. William Pancoast had secretly implanted the wife of an infertile couple with the sperm of a medical student. The student-turned-physician revealed the incident decades later, claiming it as the first case of artificial insemination, which it probably was not, but it was certainly the first *published* account.[20] Unfortunately, although the husband knew Dr. Pancoast had not used his sperm, the wife did not. News of the successful event in 1909 caused outrage (not because the wife had been deceived but because of the "unnaturalness" of the activities).

It took many decades before this type of insemination was acceptable. That is not very progressive. Had these physicians *paid* their sperm donors, their critics would have been legion. At the end of the twentieth century, AID is considered so normal that its practice is hardly mentioned, much less considered a moral issue. U.S. couples and single women can select sperm from about four hundred sperm banks, where donors are paid about $50 per donation.

Even with AID, the puritanical legacy continues, so painfully slow is progress in reproductive choice. Some "advanced" countries, like France, where the political Left's hostility toward U.S. technology has combined with religious opposition to reproductive choice, have made it illegal for single women to obtain sperm. Conservative ethicist Daniel Callahan approves of the French system, arguing that the U.S. practice devalues fatherhood.[21]

The root view here is that there should only be one way to be a father, a mother, or a family. This way is the most primitive way that has evolved so far in human evolution, which is labeled "God's way." Deviations are bad for the identity of children, bad for parents, bad for families, and devastating for society.

Perhaps the least-known and most fascinating aspect of the operation of sperm banks is that the freezing and storing of sperm involves considerable selection among sperm-donors. As the author of an overview states,

> In reality, there is a great variability between men in the post-thaw quality of their sperm. Although some sperm from most men will survive thawing, the actual efficiency of the process is less than satisfactory in regard to having fertile thawed material suitable for cervical or intrauterine insemination. A primary function of a human sperm bank currently is to recruit donors who have "freezable" sperm, namely, about 1 in every 10 men interested in being a sperm donor.[22]

What this means is that sperm banks, which have been operating for decades, are only used to create humans from that 10 percent of males whose sperm can survive freezing and thawing. Exactly what genes and phenotypes are associated with having such sperm is a matter of conjecture (in 1999, English AR clinics began to import sperm from Danish men to get better results).[23]

In sum, at first people were scared because AID sundered the creation of children from the sex act, and they probably feared that such creations would generalize too rapidly, harm the children created, and harm the institution of the family by creating children of unknown genetic fathers. None of these fears was based in fact: sex was too much fun and babies were created too easily for AID ever to become a common practice. Moreover, it is difficult to see how babies could be harmed by being created via AID, since (1) they never otherwise would have existed, (2) they are as normal as babies created sexually, and (3) they are born to families who want them very much. In short, it's silly to fear that the institution of the family can be harmed by a new way of creating families.

Our second lesson from this story, an important one, is that payment for sperm over the past decades has had little impact on anything. It did not "com-modify human life" or rapidly lead to payment for other forms of creating human life.

BUYING IVF SERVICES: A GREAT MEDICAL SUCCESS STORY

A lot has happened in reproductive medicine since Louise Brown's 1978 birth. The first successful egg transfer to produce a pregnancy was done by Carl Woods in Australia in 1983 (five years later, however, egg transfer from younger women to older women was still experimental and infrequent). During the 1980s, other new methods of increasing fertility were discovered, for example, gamete intrafallopian transfer (GIFT), which unites sperm and egg not in a petri dish but inside a fallopian tube—approximately where normal conception takes place[24] (the Roman Catholic Church condones GIFT while banning IVF, for reasons that are unclear).

By the 1990s, egg retrieval no longer required surgery; it could be done by tubal aspiration, using ultrasound imaging. Also, embryos were now inserted, if at all possible, in one of the fallopian tubes, rather than in the uterus. Researchers also began doing more and more with less: a Belgian group in 1993 succeeded in using a single sperm to fertilize an egg, a process called "intracytoplasmic sperm injection" (ICSI).[25] Within a few days of the announcement of ICSI, it was being done in an AR clinic in Birmingham, Alabama, and elsewhere—such was the efficiency of these clinics in offering the newest and best services.

As a result of these early AR techniques, between 1978 and 1998 at least fifty thousand babies were born in the United States and as many as five hundred thousand babies have been born worldwide.[26] The very wanted children who are the embodied flesh of these statistics have created incalculable human happiness. Yet if one goes back and reads the early alarmist stories about the medical developments that allowed these children to be created, one senses only dread and apprehension (as in the next chapter, when we confront the typical dread about genetic enhancement).

Unfortunately, stories about new ways to choose to be mothers just aren't as exciting as stories about reproductive technology gone wild or about male conspiracies to force women into gestational bondage. Out of the thousands of physicians and staff specializing in reproductive medicine in more than four hundred clinics, only two have been found to have acted in a less than a professional manner (or perhaps more accurately, only two have been caught).[27]

On the other hand, during most of the 1990s, about 80 percent of the couples who tried IVF, spending at least $10 thousand and up to $100 thousand, still went home without a baby. In 1995, only about 19 percent of the attempts at assisted reproduction produced a healthy, take-home baby.[28] Chances are worse for women over forty. And the likelihood of success decreased with each attempt, from 13 percent on the first try to 4 percent on the fourth.[29]

In the second half of the 1990s, a spectacular development in the United States began to change these dismal rates and make IVF more efficient: namely, the use of eggs from younger women. In the fifteen years between Carl Woods's first egg transfer in 1983 and 1998, things had changed greatly: by 1998, about six thousand patients had given birth to babies who had been conceived using eggs obtained from young women.[30] Under these circumstances, the chances of taking a baby home were higher—about 30 percent—and more important, *the chances were 30 percent regardless of the age of the gestator*, making egg donation the hope of last resort for many infertile couples.

Previously, it was thought that the age of the sperm or the age of the gestational mother was the key cause of infertility. However, it turns out that although these two factors contribute, they can be overcome. The real absolute barrier to successful conception and implantation appears to be the age of the egg, with rapid drop-offs in eggs of women over age forty.

With younger eggs, however, things are different. The sperm of older men can be used, and women over forty can still gestate embryos created from eggs of younger women, giving the gestational mother a biological connection to the child. No wonder these discoveries account for the recent phenomenon of recruiting young women who will allow their eggs to be transferred to infertile, older women.

In October 1997, the first birth of a baby who had been conceived using human eggs that had been frozen occurred at an Atlanta AR clinic run by Bruce Tucker.[31] Four months later, the world first heard about a birth resulting from use of a frozen human embryo. In 1990, two embryos were created from different eggs at a California clinic.[32] One was implanted and became a baby; the other remained frozen. Seven and a half years later, the second embryo was implanted and became a male fraternal twin to his seven-year-old brother. Researchers said to them this occurrence was really quite ordinary. While the California story was being discussed, the Pennsylvania Hospital in Philadelphia said a baby had been born there the previous December, who had grown from an embryo that had been frozen for nearly eight years (they had not called a press conference because they had regarded it as no big deal).

As with freezing and thawing of sperm for AID, freezing and thawing of embryos is also implicitly a screening process because most embryos do not survive this process with the capacity to be successfully implanted. So some screening is going on, just as it is in normal, sexual reproduction, where 40 to 60 percent of embryos fail to implant in the uterus.[33]

FINANCING AR

The question of public finance of AR is highly controversial. A typical couple may pay $20 thousand to $30 thousand for several attempts at IVF (as compared with intrauterine insemination in conjunction with fertility drugs, which can cost as little as $1 thousand per attempt).

In 1998, only a few states required insurance companies to cover AR procedures.[34] For the most part, AR is a cash-and-carry (hopefully!) affair. Those who argue for public finance claim that infertility is a disease that should be subsidized by public monies like any other disease covered by medical insurance.

The public seems to believe that AR services are too expensive to fund carte blanche for everyone. Similar conclusions have been reached about the impotence-treating drug, Viagra, and about Minoxidil for male-pattern baldness, even though all these medical breakthroughs treat legitimate problems. There is the problem that once a procedure is publicly financed, the service or drug will be sought not only by people who *need* them but also by people who merely *want* them.

Gradually, people are realizing that neither government nor group medical coverage can provide each new medical service equally to everyone. Even Australians realize this. Everyone is gradually realizing that a two-tiered system, where everyone gets a basic minimum and those with more money can buy extras, is not unjust.

One benefit of the private financing of AR is that it customarily makes people think about paying for AR as a personal issue. After all, how you spend your own money is your own business. In countries such as Australia, where AR services are financed by that country's national medical system, the problems are different. Some disabled people there have argued that new developments in AR should not go forward until better services have been made available for people with disabilities. In Australia, resources are perceived as a finite pie, where a bigger slice to one means a smaller slice to another.

COMPENSATING EGG DONORS

What the press has played up and what religious conservatives object to is that egg transfer usually involves the payment of money to the young donor. This practice is called "egg donation," and the younger women typically receive fifteen hundred to three thousand dollars per donation. A guideline issued in 1993 by the American Society for Reproductive Medicine (ASRM) suggested a standard fee of twenty-five hundred dollars.

One reason money is paid for egg donation is that the process of retrieving an egg is much more complicated than that for recovering sperm. The proposed donor is required to take drugs daily for a month or more to induce superovulation, after which eggs are aspirated with a long thin needle inserted through the vagina into an ovary and guided by ultrasound imaging. According to one donor, each time an egg is sucked from an ovary, "it feels like someone kicked you there."[35] Some people claim that the drugs used increase the woman's overall lifetime risk of some cancers, although a review of the evidence in 1999 failed to confirm this claim.[36]

Critics, of course, believe that the term *egg donor* masks the essential nature of the transaction, which is the sale of a human egg. Critics worried that the traditional fiduciary relationship between physician and patient would not apply to egg donors. Surprisingly, a recent study found that donors were treated better than they expected by physicians, and that sharing experiences on the Internet served to empower egg donors.[37]

Two well-publicized advertisements (*ads*, not cases!) put critics into a froth: In the winter of 1998, a New Jersey AR clinic advertised that it would pay young women $5 thousand for one cycle of eggs (drugs inducing superovulation can produce many eggs, as the McCaughey septuplet case taught us).

The second ad ran in 1999, in a newspaper at Princeton and other Ivy League Universities, indicating that an anonymous couple was offering $50 thousand for a "woman over 6 feet tall and with SAT scores over 1450 who was willing to sell her eggs."[38] The conjunction of the amount of the money, the targeted campuses, and the desire for two specific qualities made the ad a subject of national news. A spate of articles appeared across the country in venues ranging from the *New York Times* to the *Bioethics Examiner of the University of Minnesota Center for Bioethics* to *Boston Magazine* and *The New Yorker*. Every one presented the information to the public in language that was condemnatory and sensationalistic, leaving the impression that paid assisted reproduction was an out-of-control juggernaut. Typical was the blurb beginning the article in *Boston Magazine*: "Ivy League coeds have been offered as much as $50,000 to 'donate' their eggs to infertile women. When one desperate couple bought another woman's eggs, they entered a brave new world of egg harvesting, where biology, technology, and the marketplace collide, raising disturbing questions about breeding for perfection and profit."[39]

In late October 1999, a Los Angeles photographer caused a worldwide media sensation by offering the eggs of good-looking women on an Internet site. The resemblance of this site to a pornography site, and his attempt to "auction" the eggs, fueled the sensationalism. (He may have accomplished his goal, getting publicity that otherwise would have cost him millions of dollars.) Although this offer may well have been distasteful, and although anyone bidding so exclusively on looks has obviously not learned the lesson of the Baby M case (the Sterns picked Mary Beth Whitehead to be their surrogate because she *looked* like Elizabeth Stern and ignored the fact that Mary Beth had been rejected at another agency when she said she would have difficulty giving up any child she carried), "distasteful" is not the same thing as immoral. Besides, do we want to ban good-looking young women from marrying much older, ugly, rich old men?

More than seventeen hundred other babies were created in the previous year from similar, compensated egg donations from young women.[40] Nevertheless, the way these issues are described by reporters and bioethicists on television is so commonplace that my seventy-five-year-old mother has learned to mimic them. You don't need to be a professional writer or have a Ph.D. to write about bioethics in this sensational way (most undergraduates write this way, too).

One of our pressing ethical issues is whether the market should govern the transfer of human sperm and eggs and if not, how much government should regulate it to protect prospective parents. If the prospect of young women being paid very high prices for their eggs is too much for us to bear (although we accept millions a year being paid to professional male athletes), the American Society for Reproductive Medicine or the government might have to set a fee for all such compensated egg transfers. However, numerous problems can be created by doing so, probably cumulatively worse than the problem the price setting might solve.

Perhaps we should recall in this context that, were fees not paid to the scientists and physicians who worked hard to create breakthroughs in assisted reproduction, few of those American babies created by AR would now exist. Can we imagine very many young women voluntarily going through egg donation just for altruistic reasons? These issues are similar to issues brought up in the debates previously discussed about plasmapheresis, blood donation, kidney donation, and bone marrow donation, as well as to those raised in the debate over paid surrogate mothers (coming up soon).

The major problem here is that if you don't permit monetary compensation, you don't get young eggs and, hence, you don't get the babies that people want. If you compromise and permit compensation but not a market, other problems arise.

For example, in April 1998, the New York State Task Force on Life and Law issued a *Report on Assisted Reproductive Technologies,* and attempted to have it both ways—payment, but neither too much nor too little.[41] This committee came up with a reasonable position that reflected an ethics-by-compromise position. (Unfortunately, the recommendation won't stand the test of time.)

The approach they adopted in suggesting a set fee mirrors the dangers of central planning in socialist countries such as Cuba and China. The fee is supposed to reimburse donors for their time and effort, not for their eggs. Since the time required and pain endured for egg donation should be roughly the same for every donor, the commissioners reasoned, it should be easy to set a standard fee for all donors. In this way, they hoped to avoid the bidding up of eggs from certain women with qualities deemed to be desirable.

In practice, however, this solution leaves everyone attempting to do what bureaucrats in planned countries have never been able to do: understand all the complexities of human beings and set a price reflecting what they believe a given service "should" sell for. If such a fee is set too low, too few will accept it, but if it is set too high, too few will pay for it.

The commissioners were forced into this box because they didn't want the fee to be set so low that is was "exploitative" of poor women or so high that it was "coercive" of the same. They are thus in the business of gazing into crystal balls and second-guessing the inner springs that move women to do reproductive work. They are also mistakenly assuming that the same fee will be "exploitative" or "coercive" for all women—an obvious falsehood. In this regard, the complicated reasons women have for engaging in such new "reproductive work" need more careful examination.

Like Australians and like some critics of rewarded cadaveric donation, the New York commissioners put themselves in a box by worrying about whether AR services would be equally available to all women. This is like banning certain women from working on a Mercedes assembly line because they will never be able to afford such a car. Should we also ban women from working as nannies unless they can afford a nanny themselves?

As with paid organ donation, there is a frustrating tendency for people to pick on new reproductive options to express their vague egalitarian intuitions. But we always need to ask, not just of new reproductive advances but of any new medical advance, why should it be made available equally to all? There is a distressing lack of understanding among many people that it is possible for a medical system to be just without subsidizing equal benefits to all.

As with paying for blood and rewarded organ donation, the English and Europeans love to criticize U.S. commercialism and exaggerate its dangers. Mark Sauer, a leading U.S. researcher in AR, relates, "While attending the World Congress [in 1996] of in-vitro fertilization in Vienna, I was impressed by the almost universal criticism leveled at practitioners in the USA by colleagues abroad with respect to the payment of [egg] donors. Allegations of 'pimping' for patients in need of eggs seemed a rather cruel accusation."[42] Yvon Englert, a Belgian researcher was convinced that "U.S. oocyte donors come from the middle and poor classes of American society" (false, most are solidly middle class) and that, with payment, "the risks for both donors and receivers not to observe sanitary norms are much higher, oocyte donors being interested in hiding possible health problems."[43] So pervasive is Titmuss's view about the evils of payment, so accustomed are Europeans to providing medical services without any direct payment by patients, that Europeans constantly exaggerate the dangers of money. Yet all the European researchers at the above-mentioned World Congress lamented the lack of young female egg donors in their own countries and the consequent lack of children for many infertile couples!

In general, we don't want to regulate the price of something that, in truth, only a real market can correctly gauge. Whether it is worth $10 thousand or $30 thousand for a woman to be a nanny, surrogate mother, or assembly-line worker will depend on dozens of factors about each woman—factors that will change from year to year even for a particular woman. Only a variable payment will accurately reflect variable mixes of these factors.

Experience has shown that, because of the travail involved, too few people will come forth to offer the human tissue or services necessary to create or sustain human life if they are not paid. How much it is necessary to pay will depend on many factors. (As one of my female medical students told me, "I would do it for $50 thousand, but certainly not for $5 thousand.") If one accepts the premise that creating wanted human life is a primary good, if one believes that choice about such lives should be up to humans, and if one believes that people will respond differentially based on the amount offered, then society should allow unregulated payment for such services.

For the sake of efficiency, and this is an empirical claim, we should let the market decide how much is enough for any particular woman. Unlike in paying for organs removed from cadavers, preset fees will not work well with egg donors. This is not just a moment-in-time transaction, but a transaction that out of necessity must occur over time, as the egg donor takes drugs to superovulate and works with the adopting couple, often over many months if the first attempt is unsuccessful. *Hundreds of hours of work can be involved in such transactions.* As such, the money paid is just one factor among many in the complex relationship among egg donor, adopting couple, and AR staff. It will take differing amounts of money to motivate different women to do all that is required.

SELECTING TRAITS IN THE MARKET

At some AR clinics, extra eggs are stored to be used for infertile couples. Pictures of the women from whom the eggs were taken are available to be shown to prospective parents, and indeed, private egg brokers may arrange a meeting between prospective buyers and sellers.[44]

Some critics argue that allowing any selection by prospective parents is wrong and that such parents should be forced to accept the first available embryo or embryos should be randomly assigned. Such procedures would likely be unacceptable to many prospective couples, however, because most want to maintain the semblance of an ordinary pregnancy and childhood, which means that they try to select an embryo from parents who will be racially and ethnically as close to them as possible.

Many infertile foreign couples come to U.S. physicians for AR either because their own countries do not offer such services or because there are few suitable egg and sperm donors in their own countries. As such, they are only interested in a very specific kind of donor, for example, Japanese-American for prospective Japanese parents.

In a small number of AR clinics in the United States, couples may select already-existing embryos at a cost ($2,750) much less than what it would cost ($16,000) to create an embryo from people selected in advance. Existing embryos are created when couples change their minds after contracting for an egg donor. When that happens, the donor has already taken fertility drugs for a month and her ovaries are full of ripe eggs, so the clinics remove the eggs and fertilize them with a variety of different sperm, keeping records of each embryo created. Couples may then select an embryo from this woman's eggs (seeing a picture and description of her) that was fertilized by sperm from a man whose picture they see and whose life they read about.

Will such choice lead to desires for only perfect babies? Although this is the topic of chapter 5, it is appropriate to mention here that the use of single-cell techniques permits screening for genetic diseases. Many people believe that it is permissible to use such techniques to let infertile couples choose *against* diseases that embryos might carry. Sensationalistic stories imply that allowing preimplantation genetic diagnosis (PID) will lead to a society that encourages eugenics. This fear and the fear that people will only desire perfect babies are baseless right now. The reason can be explained in a single fact: the cost of screening for a single disease can be as much as $20 thousand, which most insurance companies will not pay.[45] Thus, the idea that a couple will screen out hundreds of embryos and only implant the perfect one is ridiculous because few couples have the money to pay for such batches of tests. Even if cheaper methods are developed, costs of using in vitro fertilization (the only way to test embryos) will keep the costs of such testing high. In general, genetic testing is done much less frequently than current discussions imply (I will discuss other objections in chapter 5).

What worries critics is that, if couples already want to try to influence the traits of their future babies and if there is a market for sperm and egg sellers,

then couples will select traits in ways the critics don't like. That is, they will select traits of donor men and women that the purchasing couple deems desirable. As one such critic put it in discussing a market for egg donors, "this approach is harmful not only because it serves to reinforce social prejudice but
also because it fragments women as persons by commodifying their characteristics, which seems at least as harmful as commodifying their eggs."[46]

The implications of this view for denial of personal choice are staggering.
There is a whole range of choices in life where people make selections based
on what they value in others: in fraternities and sororities, in country clubs, in
hiring and firing, in dating, in choosing a person to marry and to have children
with, in making friends, and in deciding where to live. Many of those choices
will seem to critics to "reinforce social prejudice," but should all choices then
be banned or regulated by government?

Second, what is the alternative to allowing choice? A set product? Choice
only within a certain range? To do this would be like requiring people to buy
only those cars rated highly by *Consumer Reports*. There is nothing special
about choices in assisted reproduction; they are being sensationalized in ways
that our normal choices are not.

PAID SURROGATE MOTHERS

It is time to rethink the widespread opposition to commercial surrogacy. A few
sensationalized cases have created a knee-jerk "yuck" response to the idea that
gestating a baby for another woman should be paid work. The actual experience
of 99 percent of paid surrogates tells a different story. Almost all cases of purchased, reproductive assistance have happy endings for all parties, resulting in
wanted babies, and are therefore morally permissible (more on this later).

Currently, some states make commercial surrogacy illegal or make contracts
about such surrogacy unenforceable. Such laws grossly overreact to a few bad
cases, banning a practice resulting in 99 percent good because 1 percent of the
cases have gone awry. On the basis of such reasoning, marriage and creation of
children through normal sex could never be justified. It is just the newness of
the procedure and the money involved in buying reproductive help that throws
off the judgments of ordinary people.

There is an unfortunate pattern in cases involving reproductive ethics where
a lack of attention to reason, numbers, and evidence produces a skewed reaction to a few cases that are sensationalized in the national media. The Baby M
case in 1986, as well as three other overly publicized cases, caused many people to think that all cases of surrogacy end in disaster.[47] In the Baby M case,

Mary Beth Whitehead reneged on a contract to bear a child for William Stern and his wife. Forced in the first trial to hand over a child that had half her genes, Mary Beth won on appeal, getting visiting rights as the legal mother. More important, this court made illegal the kind of reproductive work that Mary Beth had contracted to do for $10 thousand.

To one side, the Baby M case showed a manipulative attempt by a disturbed woman to gain a child and to breach a contract that the law ought to have enforced. To the other side, it represented a disturbing tendency to make a commodity of human reproduction. I think both sides missed the big picture.

Now that the dust has settled a decade later, it is easier to see the Baby M case for what it was. As Nanette Dembitz, a local New Jersey judge who had seen thousands of cases in her family court, said, it was almost entirely a dispute about child custody, which in itself was nothing new and which should focus on the best interests of the child.[48]

The Baby M case wrongly skewed the typical American's view of commercial surrogacy. Far too much has been made of this one case where the parties disagreed. Commercial surrogacy should not be made illegal. Just as rewarded giving in organ donation weds reimbursement to altruism, so here we wed payment to benevolent gestation.

Whether it is a case of a couple divorcing and fighting over disposal of embryos, or a couple divorcing after hiring a surrogate mother, all these are essentially divorce cases with disputes about marital property, and there is nothing unusual—unfortunately—in that. What is different is that the "property" in dispute is human eggs, embryos, or fetuses, and the media focuses on that, while ignoring thousands of cases where human babies and children are involved—which of course is banal and not "news." What is truly sad is that all these cases are just disputes by ordinary people over custody and divorce.

Some critics claim that paying for gestation is wrong because it commercializes something that a woman should do for love. This argument hits the issue of monetary payment hard. Presumably, altruistic surrogacy would be permissible, but when money is paid, women are gestating children for the wrong reasons.

This objection stems partly from romanticism about childbearing and partly from a view that what women do biologically is their natural fate, not something they should be paid for. This is the problem with the regulatory impulse, for once we decide to regulate, we set a higher goal than we will accept in unregulated practices.[49]

If instead we were to conceptualize attempts to get pregnant and the subsequent gestation of a child as real work for a woman over a year, then the question Why *shouldn't* she be paid for such work? would arise. Certainly a man would want to be paid. Whatever men do—be it sports, missionary work, or political lobbying—they deem important and expect payment for doing it. Whenever possible, employers will try to get women to do the same work for less pay or even for no pay ("Let's get some volunteers to hand out those flyers!").

The view that altruistic surrogacy is okay but commercial surrogacy is not parallels the view that organs should only be donated out of altruism, not for money. We accept selfish or mixed motives in most ordinary situations in life, but then become aghast when the same motives are present in novel situations. We too frequently posit an idealized view of human nature for legal and public policy that is more frequently falsified than instantiated.

Anthropologist Helena Ragone enlightened us on this topic by interviewing women who had worked as surrogates. Her findings contain surprises, just as the facts of real life often surprise a priori reasoning in ethics.[50] She interviewed twenty-eight women during 1988–1990, who had been surrogates in established programs. "Established" contrasted with part-time programs run by physicians, lawyers, and adoption agencies. During hundreds of hours of formal interviews, Ragone spoke not only with these twenty-eight women who had worked as surrogates but also with seventeen individual members of couples who had hired surrogates.[51]

Studying such women from the perspective of kinship theory, Ragone wondered how they saw their roles and adjusted to the widespread social perception of them as "deviant mothers" or "rent-a-womb" women. Surprisingly, most surrogates were already mothers and saw themselves in altruistic ways. The money allowed them to be employed in what they saw as their natural, God-given role: to create life, to be mothers, to help others. This is a classic case of people having mixed motives and creating good results.

The most astounding conclusions drawn by Ragone have far-reaching implications. Far from destroying the family, paid surrogacy actually creates family in two important senses. First, being a surrogate allowed these mothers to stay at home with their own children, to "be there for them," in contrast with other employment that would require the women to leave home and either use day care or leave latchkey children at home alone.

Second, of course, the woman is offering the "gift of life" to an infertile couple. The surrogates were well aware that they were giving something special to the other couple—something that went beyond the money they were being paid.

The other surprising result was that the surrogates didn't mind giving up the baby—unlike in the Baby M case—but had trouble ceasing the intimacy that had evolved with the adoptive couple. The surrogates also experienced some sadness upon ending the role of pregnant mother and giving up the feeling of being special to everyone because of it.

This sadness confirms a widely reported result discovered by nurse-researcher Nancy Reame, who interviewed ten surrogates who had given birth a decade before. Six of the ten expressed some disappointment, not at having been surrogates but because the "relationship had been abandoned by the adoptive couple at the time of birth (for 3 women) or over time (for 3 women)."[52] The disappointed six expected long-term contact with the adoptive couple, that is, they expected a continuation of their sense of being extremely special to the couple as life-giver. These expectations, of course, were unrealistic.

The most important point here is that we should think of surrogacy as real work, not as a perversion of motherhood. Think of it not as a woman being paid to give up "her" baby, but as an innovative way of paying women who have a natural talent for gestation. As one surrogate said, "I love being pregnant and I didn't want to raise another child. I have easy pregnancies."[53]

Another common objection to paid surrogacy is that it's wrong because it's not best for the child. This objection holds that it's wrong to deliberately bring a child into the world where the gestational work is not performed by the rearing mother. Paying for gestation is inherently wrong, because a child created this way who will likely have a confused identity with at least three, and maybe five (should divorce enter the picture), parents will be harmed.

As time passes, I think we will come to see this objection as the same as saying that it's wrong for a woman to have a child whom she doesn't rear herself and instead uses day care, public schools, and baby-sitters to do the work for her. Wealthy families in past centuries and today have nannies and au pairs who do the real work of day-to-day child raising. Long ago, we handed over home schooling to professional teachers. Whether such arrangements are best for the child largely depends on the details of the case and the motives of the parties involved. Properly done, such arrangements need not be bad for the child.

Such concerns raise the question of whether children created by AID or anonymous egg donation or gestated by surrogates can be harmed by not knowing the characteristics of their genetic ancestors and by being barred from ever having a relationship with these ancestors. One compromise nicely solves this problem: allow (don't require) gametic donors or surrogates to be confidential but not anonymous. In this practice, the names and identities of donors are kept from children created from gametes, but these men and women are allowed (or encouraged) to update their files every five to ten years, so that their biological children can know about genetic diseases and their lives. This practice protects the desire of some donors and some surrogates not to have contact with children created from their gametes, while also giving them the chance to change their minds.

Perhaps surprisingly, many sperm and egg donors, or surrogates, do not mind maintaining such records and express a desire to know about the lives of the children they helped produce.[54] It is mainly the parents who pay for the donated sperm, egg, or embryo or adopt the child who object to the children knowing the donors.[55] Thus, making the sharing of such knowledge optional would not tend to discourage people from donating sperm and eggs or from being surrogates and would allow the children to find out who else created them and why.

A third objection says that paying for gestation is wrong because it exploits women. This argument is really about the amount of money paid, not about the act of paying money. Sometimes it masquerades as an objection to commercialization. The mask is lifted when one asks, "Well, then, just how much would a surrogate have to be paid in order for it NOT to be considered exploitation?" If the interlocutor cannot come up with a sum, then the true objection surfaces.

The catch-22 faced by the New York State Task Force in trying to navigate these waters by regulating payment for eggs can be illustrated another way, using surrogacy as the example. Suppose someone suggests that paying a surrogate a million dollars would surely disqualify such an arrangement from being categorized as exploitative. But people would then object, "That is such a large amount of money that it distorts the arrangement. People shouldn't be tempted so strongly to commercialize something private and personal." In this case, the proponent of commercialization can't win at any amount—be it low or high!

Sometimes, this objection also implies that surrogates are being exploited by men. Certainly from reading Ragone's interviews, nothing could be further from the truth. Paid surrogacy seems to almost universally empower the women who do it, making them feel special and like they're contributing real money to their family's income. A *surrogates large number of women become surrogates despite objections from their husbands*, or must battle husbands who want to keep the baby. Ragone found no case of a woman being a surrogate who was exploited by a man.

A final objection is that, although not intrinsically wrong, paying for gestation will soon lead to exploitation of the poor by the rich. Again, this tired argument shouldn't be used to pick on surrogacy. It applies to any service that rich people can buy that poor people can't. It ignores that some middle-class people will value a particular service so much that they will forgo normal middle-class desires in order to buy a service that "only rich people" can afford.

Indeed, whether it's paid organ donation or reproductive services, why should the argument of equity be assumed to have special force in these areas? It's not as if we have a real national policy that would achieve such equity in housing, employment, and access to medical care or public education (and aren't these issues much more important?).

Exploitation is about not having any choices. Paid surrogacy is about expanding choices for infertile couples and about expanding the definition of what society values about women. That does not sound like exploitation of women to me.

The wrong assumption here is the simplistic, either-or categorization. Indeed, perhaps the really exploitative argument would be to say that only "good," unpaid, altruistic women should be allowed to be surrogates—what is often called the "compassion trap." This is the false first step of casting all surrogates as either whores or Madonnas: either be "good" and earn no money, or be "bad" and earn money. The compassion trap also has the insidious implication that women who bear children for others for money aren't compassionate, just greedy.

In conclusion, selecting a woman to be your egg donor is not that different from selecting a woman to gestate your embryo. In both cases, there can be a long relationship between a couple and the hired woman. In both cases, the woman getting paid combines altruism with real work.

CONCLUSIONS

New changes in reproductive medicine, especially when accompanied by financial incentives, have always created stormy waters. Yet, when permitted to flourish, they have sailed along fine, creating new families and loved children. As the history of assisted reproduction shows, such developments are not evils but blessings, part of a great, modern success story of a new kind of medicine.

Payment for eggs and gestation has neither enslaved nor degraded women. If anything, it has empowered them. It recognizes and values the unique contribution of women and allows some to live as stay-at-home, traditional mothers with their own children. We must beware of simplistic, either-or conceptualizations of paid reproductive help and recognize that most people do most things for mixed motives, including contracting for reproductive services.

Paying for such reproductive help allows reproduction to happen. There is a continuum of help here, from paying for sperm to paying for gestation, and the important thing is to look at the intentions and results, not the technical means employed. If all parties want to create healthy wanted children, and that is the result, then the means used and how much the means are compensated should not be the primary moral issue, if they are "moral" issues at all.

NOTES

1. Seale Harris, *Woman's Surgeon: The Life Story of J. Marion Sims* (New York: Macmillan, 1950), 245.

2. J. Marion Sims, *Clinical Notes on Uterine Surgery* (New York: J. H. Vail, 1886).

3. Margaret Marsh and Wanda Ronner, *The Empty Cradle: Infertility in America from Colonial Times to the Present* (Baltimore, Md.: Johns Hopkins University Press, 1996), 72.

4. Harris,*Woman's Surgeon,* 308.

5. Marsh and Ronner, *The Empty Cradle,* 73.

6. "Internet Offers Embryos by Mail," *Herald Sun* (Melbourne, Australia), 10 May 1988, 2.

7. Ibid.

8. Christopher Hill, *The World Turned Upside Down: Radical Ideas during the English Revolution* (New York: Penguin, 1972), 312–13.

9. Stephanie Coontz, *The Way We Never Were* (New York: Basic Books, 1992), 11–12.

10. Ibid., 227.

11. Ibid., 227ff.

12. Joana Levy, "Conservatives Clash with Psychologists," *Birmingham Post-Herald,* 23 August 1999, C4.

13. Ronald Green, "Human Embryo Research: What Are the Issues?" *The Lahey Clinic Medical Ethics Newsletter* (Spring 1998), 1.

14. Maggie Scarf, "The Fetus as Guinea Pig," *New York Times Magazine,* 19 October 1975, 194–200.

15. Ibid.

16. Paul Ramsey, *The Ethics of Fetal Research* (New Haven, Conn.: Yale University Press, 1975), 89.

17. "Blair's Blunder," *New Scientist,* 3 July 1999, 3.

18. Harris, *Woman's Surgeon,* 246–8.

19. Ibid.

20. Elaine Tyler May, *Barren in the Promised Land: Childless Americans and the Pursuit of Happiness* (Cambridge, Mass.: Harvard University Press, 1995), 65–9.

21. John Leo, "Sperm Banks Promote Fatherlessness," *Birmingham News,* 9 May 1995.

22. Armand M. Karow, "Implications of Tissue Banking for Human Reproductive Medicine," in *Reproductive Tissue Banking: Scientific Principles,* ed. A. Karow and John Critser (San Diego, Calif.: Academic Press, 1977), 444.

23. "The Viking Baby Invasion," *Mail* (London), Internet site, 10 October 1999.

24. Glenn Kramon, "Infertility Chain: The Good and Bad in Medicine," *New York Times,* 19 June 1992, C1.

25. Gina Kolata, "New Pregnancy Hope: A Single Sperm Injected," *New York Times,* 11 August 1993, B7.

26. "Miracle Babies," *People* (21 October 1998): 62.

27. Cecil Jacobson of Fairfax, Virginia, was indicted in 1991 on fifty-three counts of fraud and perjury for using his own sperm to create embryos; he went to jail. Ricardo Asch, from southern California, fled to South America after implanting Debbie Callender's embryos in another woman's womb without Callender's consent.

28. Sheryl Gay Stolberg, "For the Infertile, a High-Tech Treadmill of Despair," *New York Times,* Internet site, 14 December 1997.

29. Centers for Disease Control, "Assisted Reproductive Technology Success Rates in the United States: 1996 National Summary and Fertility Clinic Reports" (CDC Web site).

30. Sheryl Gay Stolberg, "Quandary on Donor Eggs: What to Tell the Children," *New York Times,* Internet site, 18 January 1998.

31. Gina Kolata, "Successful Births Reported with Frozen Human Eggs," *New York Times*, 17 October 1997, A1.

32. David Colker, "It's a Boy—Embryo Is Viable after 1990 Freezing," *Los Angeles Times*, 17 February 1998.

33. A. Wilcox et al., "Incidence of Early Loss of Pregnancy," *New England Journal of Medicine* 319, no. 4 (28 July 1988): 189–94.

34. Stolberg, "For the Infertile."

35. "Egg Donation," *60 Minutes*, 2 October 1994.

36. *BioNews*, 19 October 1999, reporting on results announced at the annual meeting of American Society for Reproductive Medicine, 16th World Congress on Fertility and Sterility, American Society of Reproductive Medicine 54th Annual Meeting (San Francisco), 5 October 1988.

37. Andrea Kalfoglou and Gail Geller, "Navigating the Conflict of Interest in Oocyte Donation," presented 29 October 1999 at the Philadelphia meeting of the American Society for Bioethics and Humanities.

38. Gina Kolata, "Soaring Price of Donor Eggs Sets Off Debate," *New York Times*, 25 February 1998, A1; Adrienne Knox, "Brokers and Fertility Clinics in Bidding War for Women Willing to Sell Eggs from Ovaries," *Birmingham News*, 15 March 1998, A3.

39. Lisa Gerson, "Human Harvest," *Boston Magazine* (May 1999): 106.

40. So said a spokesperson for the American Society for Reproductive Medicine on the *Today Show* on 25 October 1999.

41. New York State Task Force on Life and Law, *Report on Assisted Reproductive Technologies* (Albany, N.Y.: 1998).

42. Mark Sauer, "Ooycte Donation: Reflections on Past Work and Future Directions," *Human Reproduction* 11, no. 6 (1996): 1150.

43. Yvon Englert, "Ethics of Oocyte Donation Is Challenged by the Nature of the Health System." Commentary on Mark Sauer, above, in *Human Reproduction*.

44. Gina Kolata, "With Help of Science, Infertile Couples Can Even Pick Traits," *New York Times*, 23 November 1997, A1.

45. Frederic Golden, "Good Eggs, Bad Eggs," *Time* (11 January 1999): 58.

46. Mary Rutz, "Selling Eggs: Cost and Consent in the Bull Market," *Bulletin of the University of Illinois at Chicago Department of Medical Education* 5, no. 2 (January 1999): 3.

47. These are the 1986 Baby M case, the Malahoff case (where it was revealed on the *Donahue Show* that Alexander Malahoff wasn't the father), a Tennessee case, where a drug-using surrogate tried to blackmail the adoptive couples, the *Johnson v. Calvert* case in California, where a black nurse gestated the embryo created from the egg and sperm of a white couple, then changed her mind about giving up the baby, and the "Jaycee" case in California, where a child was successfully gestated from a donor egg and sperm, but the couple hiring the surrogate divorced after the gestation began.

48. Nanette Dembitz, quoted by Vivian Cadden, "Hard Questions about the Baby M Case," *McCall's* (June 1985): 58.

49. I owe this point and several others in this chapter to the great work of Kelly Smith in reviewing this book.

50. Helena Ragone, *Surrogate Motherhood: Conception in the Heart* (Boulder, Colo.: Westview Press, 1994), 67.

51. Ibid., 4–6.

52. Nancy Reame, "Surrogate Mothers Feel Disappointment," presented at the 16th World Congress on Fertility and Sterility, American Society of Reproductive Medicine 54th Annual Meeting (San Francisco), 5 October 1988.

53. Ragone, *Surrogate Motherhood*, 61.

54. Cynthia Cohen, "Parents Anonymous," *Egg Donation*, ed. Cynthia Cohen (Baltimore, Md.: Johns Hopkins University Press, 1997).

55. Sheryl Gay Stolberg, "Quandary on Donor Eggs: What to Tell the Children," *New York Times*, 18 January 1998, A13.

5

RE-CREATING CHILDREN: CHOOSING TRAITS

I have spread my dreams under your feet:
Tread softly.

—William Butler Yeats,
"He Wishes for the Cloths of Heaven"

To Our Descendants in a Far-off Time,

In the year 2010, we write this letter to you. We do not expect the time capsule into which it has been put to be opened for many centuries. We write to explain to you the decisions we are making now about genetic screening and enhancement that will affect who you are. We hope to illustrate the ethical disagreements of our time and to show you how difficult it is for us to change.

Who are we? We are parents, children of parents, aunts, uncles, teachers, physicians, mail workers, shipbuilders, Internet designers, writers, athletes, businesspeople, and government officials. What we had in common was a desire that the future be better, but our desire was not for some abstract future, but for *your* future.

As we write this letter, advances in medical genetics can give parents better choices about the kinds of children they have, but at the same time, dark clouds loom on the horizon. Leaders in government, academia, religion, bioethics, and Hollywood want to limit choice.

The most important thing we are doing is giving parents *permission* to choose better kids. Many parents are worried about being criticized for wanting "perfect kids" when they bring up the subject with their family physicians (genetic counselors never became widespread, partly because reimbursement for their services was hard to create and partly because people trusted their physicians more).

When cheap multitesting kits for embryos became available in 2007, it became easy and inexpensive to test for more than a hundred genetic diseases, and critics raised the familiar "perfect baby" fear. Nevertheless, few parents in fact have chosen to use such tests, mainly because of widely publicized cases where embryos repeatedly tested positive for different genetic diseases through three or four pregnancies (resulting in early abortions in each case). The best way to assure a normal pregnancy has been through in vitro fertilization, creation of multiple embryos, and preimplantation testing, but that is still too expensive, cumbersome, and inefficient for most parents.

Hence, embryo screening and its resulting legacy to future members of this genetic line only affects the 1 percent of the population trying to avoid hereditary, lethal genetic diseases (and seeking coverage for preventive genetic tests) and another 1 percent trying to give their kids the best genetic base. The other 98 percent of citizens of developed countries, and 99.99 percent of people on the planet, are unaffected.

These facts are not generally well understood. Most people still want to restrict choice for those seeking the best genetic base for their kids.

Your fate carries a lot of weight with us because we are utilitarians: we are six billion, ten generations of you will be *sixty, seventy, or possibly eighty billion*. How can we *not* try to improve your lives? In our better moments, we know there is so much more to come after us—so many kisses, so many happy births, so many new great novels, so many great medical discoveries. (Perhaps genetic medicine will even bring a better sense of humor, especially about bioethics—wouldn't that be wonderful?)

As we write, we have no crystal ball to see into the future. Whatever happens, keep in mind one truth. As we choose, many values and interests compete for our allegiance. Some people want to protect the status quo, to preserve the traditional family, to make society strictly egalitarian, or to never take any risks at all. Throughout all the discussions, our one guiding question is this: What's in the best interest of the people to come? It doesn't matter what parents want, what society wants, or what the current fashion is. What matters is what is best for "our grandkids to come," for you.

THE INTERGENERATIONAL ASSEMBLY

Believe it or not, you already exist for us. We imagine you and dozens of other, future generations coming together with us in a big assembly with the goal of deciding what a just, democratic society permits for improving future children.

In doing so, we borrow from philosopher, John Rawls, whose theory of justice calls such an assembly "the original position." To make choice just here, Rawls stipulates that it must be under a "veil of ignorance" where we cannot know our race, gender, personal wealth, health, age, sexual orientation, or any other morally arbitrary, personal fact about ourselves. In one passage, Rawls discusses intergenerational, genetic justice under this veil of ignorance: "it is also in the interest of each to have greater natural assets. . . . The pursuit of reasonable policies in this regard *is something that earlier generations owe to later ones,* this being a question that arises between generations"[1] (our emphasis). This passage galvanized us, because we started out just looking for *permission* to improve future generations and here Rawls argues that we are *obligated* to do so.

If we imagine ourselves with you in such a huge assembly, then when the veil is lifted, we will not know in which generation we will be: we could be in the sorry state of the present, with genetic diseases and genotypes decreed by the spin of the genetic roulette wheel, or we could be in some far better body and mind developed by, say, the year 2600. If we then ask, "What kind of mind and body do we want, to the extent that these can be controlled by genetic choices over generations?" the answer is clear: we want a body free of the dangerous genetic diseases, a body that can function well for at least a hundred years, intelligence and good memory, and a personality that is disposed to be happy. Life is better when it starts this way.

Indeed, suppose we are able to give you such qualities but deliberately held them back (perhaps because we resent you living happier lives), wouldn't you judge us immoral? Wouldn't you think we had harmed you by choosing to have you lack what you could have had? It would be as if Prozac became owned by Scientologists, who decided that ordinary people would "grow more" by suffering through depression and anxiety and thus withheld the drug.

Rawls's veil of ignorance, applied intergenerationally to the future, forces us to apply the Golden Rule to decisions about your qualities. As time crawls without society making any decisions, we realize that even decisions *not* to choose, to do nothing, have moral implications, perhaps as great as failed attempts to make you better. We realize that, even though you didn't exist, decisions we make or don't make will cross generations in both harmful and beneficial ways.

In other words, just as many *moral* issues are at stake in delaying decisions as in making them. This realization gives us a sense of urgency.

So we begin to think about how we can actually help parents choose better kids. Of course, we know that we can never make parents feel that they are *compelled* to choose a certain way. We know about the abuses and bad science during the eugenics movement in the United States at the start of the twentieth century and certainly don't want to repeat that fiasco.

AN EXAMPLE

We do not have to go into the future to find an example of how kids can be harmed by doing nothing and letting "nature take its course." In our time, a new kind of somatic genetic therapy came about for children of Mennonite and Amish couples with Crigler-Najjar syndrome. In this condition, a crucial enzyme is lacking that allows the liver to remove bilirubin, a toxic by-product of the body. As bilirubin accumulates, the skin of such patients becomes jaundiced. Without genetic therapy, children with Crigler-Najjar syndrome must spend ten to twelve hours a day in a mirrored bed with lights that break down the bilirubin. The children hate sleeping this way, and the therapy loses its effectiveness as the children become adults, but the alternative is death.

A new form of genetic therapy, chimeraplasts, was first tried in 2000 on Crigler-Najjar patients. The therapy stimulated the genes to repair the damage they all shared at a single point mutation. The therapy was partially successful, and with liver transplants later for adults, allowed most patients to live to mid-adulthood. The media of the time hailed this as a great success.

From our point of view, it was a gigantic failure, for the disease needn't have existed in the first place if the parents and community had been more responsible. The seventy-five thousand sect members in Lancaster County, Pennsylvania, were descended from just forty-seven original families. Because young men and women of the "Plain People" (as the Amish and Mennonites call themselves) were forbidden to marry outside their sects, children of these marriages had a high rate of inherited diseases such as Crigler-Najjar. In the year 2000, sixteen children had this disease in Lancaster County alone.

The tragedy was that all these cases were preventable. By using family trees and genealogy maps, by testing adults for the genes they carry, and by doing preimplantation diagnosis (PID) in embryos when using in vitro fertilization, no Crigler-Najjar baby need have been born.

We estimated, assuming a liver transplant at some point, that it costs $1 million to treat each child with Crigler-Najjar. The genetic therapies have not

proven to be the hoped-for, one-shot "magic bullets," but are like AZT and protease inhibitors for HIV infection: complicated, ongoing treatments that halt
the progression of the disease but don't instantly eradicate it. So children suffer most of their lives, being dragged from one hospital to another, building up
a fear of people in white coats.

When we suggested in 2000 that these were "tragic births," we were called
"Nazis" and "fascists," but we were not—as our critics screamed—suggesting
mandatory abortions or desirous of making women into "breeding factories."
As said, we know all too well the painful history of the early twentieth century,
which had witnessed a horrible eugenics movement based on class prejudice,
extreme ignorance of genetics, and hatred of minorities. Worries about a
resurgence of such crude, state-influenced eugenics haunted every decision
we made.

Because no parent wants his or her child to be genetically cursed, people in
some communities took matters into their own hands. Tay-Sachs disease runs,
like Crigler-Najjar in the Plain People, in Ashkenazi Jewish families, and it is a
lethal genetic disease that destroys beautiful young Jewish children in their
prime. Initially, and despite the high incidence of this disease where intermar-
riage within the community was required, preventing babies with Tay-Sachs
was difficult because of opposition to abortion and the fear among carriers of
being stigmatized. But in the early 1970s, Ashkenazi Jews themselves began to
prepare over fourteen months to reduce the number of such births. The effort
began in orthodox communities in Brooklyn and used matchmakers. In the following two decades, more than a million young adults were screened, thousands of pregnancies with Tay-Sachs were terminated, and many thousands
more were prevented by not having carriers match as marriage partners.

Was this a bad "eugenic" result? Of all ethnic groups, we thought that Jewish families would be the least likely to use genetic screening for bad ends, to
create a "Master Race." Of course, they were only engaged in so-called negative eugenics, trying to eliminate disease, not positive eugenics, trying to create
better humans.

In retrospect, these ethnic traditions did create better children. So, too, did
communities originating from the Indian subcontinent, many with a long tradition of brokered marriages between large families, who quickly began genetic
screening against lethal diseases. As the Japanese and Icelanders followed, we
saw that the incidence of some genetic diseases could be reduced by strenuous,
voluntary efforts.

But governments in the United States and Europe were reluctant to change.
In the States, traditionalists exerted great leverage; and in Europe, critics on
the Left feared state-mandated eugenics. And no wonder: in our time, all the

movies, television shows, and science fiction novels warned of impending doom from expanded genetic choice.

To counterattack, we created a new position in society, modeled after the Dalai Lama. We call her, "Speaker for the Future." Her job (and so far, only women have been elected) is to be the voice for all those sixty to eighty billion people waiting in the wings of our present age's play. As only possible people at present, they have no voice but Her. The speaker's job is an onerous one, a great one, one few people would want, for she must make the weight of the future's needs felt amidst the clamor of the "now." We have become a people of a short attention span, accustomed to immediate pleasures and focused on sound bites and news update via Internet monitors everywhere. So rarely do most people think six to ten generations ahead. It is Her job to make us think that way.

FATALISM VERSUS EXPANDED GENETIC CHOICE

Our opponents argue that new genetic choices should be forbidden to parents. They are reproductive fatalists who assert that human choice is impotent and that humans should bow to this assumption: "What God has decreed, human choice cannot affect."

It is easy to see how fatalism arose from primitive times when it was foolish to expect too much of any particular child; parents then never knew what kind of child would be born or how a particular child would turn out. Theologically, one could then say it was all God's doing that a particular child was smart or not. So also, genetic disease and disability were seen as "God's will," as a "gift" with special meaning, or as deserved as punishment for sin.

But why is a random but worrisomely high chance of a problem better to accept than taking preventive measures? We could appeal to tradition, to how we've always just accepted any child who comes along, but what's so good about a tradition that has such a high cost to the children afflicted with genetic diseases?

Now, we think these old theological explanations were given after the fact to allow parents to cope with unexpected burdens. We know that genetics explains many conditions, such as the autosomal dominance of fatal diseases such as Huntington's or how breast cancer can run in families where none of the women "deserve" cancer.

Indeed, during the first two millennia the only real decision parents had to make was simply whether or not to create a child. The accepted view for centuries was that, after birth, parents needed to bond with the child and to accept responsibility for its care, not wonder about "what ifs." Indeed, part of the implicit bargain—so many said—was that in wanting a child, parents agreed to take whatever came along. (And of course, even if parents use genetic screening or try to enhance a child's capacities, the bargain is still there.)

Fatalistic attitudes made sense in past centuries when genetic medicine offered few choices. But as we write in 2010, we wonder why any couple should continue to think this way? Why should a couple be happy with any child that the flick of the genetic roulette wheel sends their way? After medicine has learned how to create better children, the appeal of fatalism seems . . . well, atavistic.

Our biggest concern was to give "ethics cover" for that 1 percent of parents who want to start their child with the best genetic base possible. Some considerations about onus of proof in public policy enter here. To date, the onus has been on parents who desire greater choice. This has been important because medical insurance plans have generally not paid for preventive genetic tests on embryos and fetuses. We are trying to reverse that.

Indeed, why shouldn't such parents be allowed to try to create the best possible child, even if critics accuse them of "playing God" and of wanting "perfect children"? If such parents want the best for their kids, why should they be shackled by well-meaning but misguided critics?

We continue to think it wrong that critics focus on preventing insurance companies from covering such genetic tests. Each year, hundreds of thousands of women conceive and gestate fetuses while high on addictive drugs, dependent on alcohol, smoking cigarettes, and working in hazardous jobs. We know pregnancy this way hurts kids, yet these same critics are reluctant to invade the "sanctity of family life" for these at-risk fetuses. They only want to take away choice for the new reproductive option, not for the old ones. All this, even though a thousand times more children are being inadvertently harmed by our tolerance of heterosexual-conception-by-drug-and-alcohol-dependent mothers than might be harmed from expanded genetic choice. Which way of reproduction harms more kids?

"GO SLOW"

We are accused of being too hasty in advocating genetic screening and more parental choice. The conventional wisdom is that we must not rush too fast into "genetic engineering," into "tampering with the gene pool," and into "changing the human history contained in our genes."

Very rarely are such thought-stopping phrases challenged. Medical ethics among physicians is very conservative and slow to change. Most professional bioethicists are also very conservative about change. Hence, advocating "go slow" is the safe, easy thing to do.

But what is the opportunity cost of going slow? How much damage is done by *not* acting, by accepting the status quo for another generation?

Take cystic fibrosis, the most common genetic disease among Caucasians (one in twenty are silent carriers, meaning they will never get the disease but one of their children might if they marry another carrier). Children with this lethal disease first present in hospitals with the "failure to thrive" syndrome and are given the "sweat test." In past decades, commercials warned parents to bring babies with salty skin to the family physician (cystic fibrosis is the only common disease that produces salty sweat in children).

As adolescents and adults, people with cystic fibrosis develop very thick secretions in their lungs. These secretions also harbor a bacterium known as psuedomonas, found only in people with cystic fibrosis. Eventually, these secretions suffocate people with cystic fibrosis.

The age of death can be delayed with treatment. Three decades ago, CF kids were dead by age three. Twenty years ago, most were dead by twenty, but by 2000, the average age at death had risen to around thirty.

One of the things that keeps some people with cystic fibrosis alive longer today is transplants of lung tissue from parents, or a whole lung transplant. (With a whole lung transplant, the person no longer has CF.)

In 2000, we knew the gene for cystic fibrosis, called the CFTR gene. More accurately, we knew that all humans have CFTR genes, but people with cystic fibrosis lack *functional* CFTR genes. Genetic therapy has to create and insert a functional CFTR gene into their systems.

Various attempts to do so were tried, using first, a nonviral approach with a plasmid surrounding a lipid, and second, using a viral vector. In the latter procedure, a crippled virus has a functional CTFR gene inserted in it, and the virus is then introduced into the lungs, usually by a nasal inhaler.

These were attempts at "somatic" gene therapy, aimed at helping only the patient with cystic fibrosis. Because such somatic therapies were not as successful as had been hoped, attempts at germ-cell (stem cell) genetic therapy were then discussed, where the CTFR gene would be inserted into the embryo or fetus. Indeed, many thought it would be easier to cure such genetic diseases with germ-line than somatic therapy. But when a patient unexpectedly died in 1999 during one experimental somatic therapy, everything got put on hold for years, not only somatic therapy but all talk of germ-line.[2]

The danger of germ-line therapy was that any bad change would also be passed on to subsequent generations. Hopefully, the only change would be the presence of a functional CTFR gene, but any unintended consequence would also be passed on. At this point, everyone said, "Go slow!"

But it was not clear why going slow is so important. Many years have gone by with somatic genetic therapy with no clear case of success. Just how many people with cystic fibrosis have to die in the name of "going slow"?

At this point, odd objections started to crop up. Scientists pointed out that any genetic disease must be in the human genome for a reason. Evolution works, after all. The same gene in blacks that causes sickle-cell anemia also protects blacks against malaria, so cystic fibrosis must also have some evolutionary function. It was speculated that the thick mucus of people with cystic fibrosis protected them against various forms of air-born plague or against the kind of lethal influenza that swept the United States around 1918. So we should be careful what we eliminate from the human genome, because there might be another flu epidemic or plague in the future.

To this objection, we retorted that there is a difference between idle speculation and practical policy. What is being suggested here? That people with cystic fibrosis not receive successful genetic therapy, that a child of maybe one in fifty must die in the prime of life, to give the human race a *possible* protection against plague and flu?

Let's suppose that cystic fibrosis did in fact give such protection and that there was great danger of such plagues and flues in the coming decades. Even so, if someone is going to save the human race by dying in his prime from cystic fibrosis, shouldn't he or she *consent*? Shouldn't they *volunteer* for this job? And if they did, shouldn't they be honored during their short lives for doing so?

Of course, once the cure is here, no one will seriously argue the above. On the other hand, while we were trying to develop a genetic cure, arguments like this were considered good arguments. Why was that? Probably because people don't think (feel) through what it means to people now who are dying from cystic fibrosis.

We have also been very slow to start genetic screening for cystic fibrosis. Given the high prevalence of silent carriers of cystic fibrosis in North America and Europe and given the lack of effective genetic therapy, why not try some model screening programs and see what happens, say, in a small state such as Delaware?

Critics have pointed out that preimplantation diagnosis (PID) is too expensive and cumbersome for such a large population. First, PID requires use of in vitro fertilization, not a very efficient procedure in the first place, and not generalizable to one in twenty Caucasians in North America. Second, if we're not using PID, we're talking about abortions, and is that what we really want to do—to encourage any family with a CF fetus to abort?

To this we replied, why not try such a screening program and see what happens? Who would have thought decades ago that Ashkenazi Jewish families would have accepted such screening? Just give the parents information: their fetus will develop cystic fibrosis as an adult, here is what that disease is like, and abortion is a legal option. In other words, use nondirective genetic counseling and see what happens.

Of course, even this very cautious approach was deemed too hasty by critics.

OUR EXPECTATIONS OF PARENTS

Historically, even twentieth-century parents tried to improve on the fickle allotments of fate: pregnant women didn't drink alcohol, parents stimulated infants (one kind of retardation is caused by boredom), didn't smoke, and ate nutritional foods. All these actions contradicted fatalistic acceptance. Children with crooked teeth got braces, those with scoliosis had steel rods implanted in their spines so they could dance through life with heads held high, and PKU kids got special diets to prevent retardation.

When it came to not physical but cognitive attributes, parental expectations were often very important. Because such cognitive attributes were seen, correctly, as malleable from an early age, society already both expected and allowed far greater parental interventions here.

Take an issue about children and parental expectations that is one of the most-contested issues of our times: public versus private schools. Although social critics blasted parents who chose private schools for their children—such critics focused more on the harm to the general population that having good kids and dedicated parents leave than on what life was like for those who stayed in public schools. And talk and printed words were cheap: what really mattered in public policy was whether such critics got enough power to *ban* parents from sending their kids to private schools.

So in the twentieth century, parents who, reading the latest studies about early formation of the brain, stayed at home during the first years of the child's life and affectionately interacted with their children, were applauded. Others sacrificed to get their children into the best schools, whether by moving to a good district or sending them to a private school. Some fathers played math games with their young daughters after dinner every night for years, with subsequent astounding SAT scores in math. And thinking about home schooling changed, as very devoted parents proved that some children educated this way outshone those educated in larger groups.

So such parents characteristically sought the best that genetic medicine had to offer. When a genetically engineered vaccine became available that prevented common viral infections, most parents wanted it for their children. When cheap genetic vaccines came along that protected against most sexually transmitted diseases, such as AIDS, hepatitis, and human papilloma virus (HPV), most parents thought they owed it to their kids to give them this "genetic leg up" against future mishap.

Consider SmartKid, a wonderful drug discovered in 2005 that enhances the foundation in the brain for memory, intelligence, and learning. SmartKid arose directly from the creation of the mentally enhanced mouse "Doogie," created in the Princeton lab of scientist Joe Z. Tsien in 1999.[3] Dr. Tsien added a gene designed to increase the speed of Doogie's brain's NMDA receptors, which governs memory and learning. Doing so made Doogie much smarter, and his increased intelligence stayed with Doogie into his mouse adulthood.

Of course, as soon as Doogie was reported, critics predicted doom and gloom. The head of the Ethics Section of the British Medical Association, Dr. Vivienne Nathanson, warned that Doogie "leads to the specter of designer babies and the concept of children being rejected because they do not have these qualities."[4] Those favoring nurture over nature suggested Tsien's results were immoral. Steven Rose, head of the brain and behavior group at the Open University in England, said, "This is a real piece of vulgar hype from Princeton. They shouldn't do this stuff; it really is irresponsible. . . . Human intelligence is something that develops as part of the interaction between children and the social and natural world, as they grow up. It is not something locked inside a little molecule in the head."[5]

Not too many parents of autistic kids adopted Rose's view when human drugs based on Doogie's results became available. SmartKid's benefits were first proven in people in 2001 with inchoate Alzheimer's, and then SmartKid was offered to children with autism and several forms of retardation. Although it did not restore normal functioning in every case, in many cases in did. Parents who had institutionalized children in despair were able to give their children SmartKid and, with increased intelligence and functioning of their brains, keep the children at home or even send them to public schools.

SmartKid had more exciting results with each new group of subjects. Its dispersal proved unstoppable. Soon kids were graduating high school knowing the world's great music, able to recite most of the world's great poetry (including gobs of Shakespeare), and speaking several foreign languages.

So obvious were the benefits that the federal government began to provide SmartKid free to the child of any parent who desired it. No parents or their children, of course, were forced to accept SmartKid, and some did not.

The effects are becoming remarkable on the workforce, propelling the economies of North America, Japan, and Iceland into great prosperity because of the brilliance of their cadres of young programmers, biotech engineers, and scientists. Indeed, it is widely debated today whether it is good to have an entire economy so dependent on teenagers, but few people think anything will change because everyone enjoys all the fruits of their discoveries and innovations.

Similar things happened with Slimline, the first genetic therapy for severely overweight people. With the change of one group of genes, such people no longer craved sweets, no longer ate to get the inner "sigh" of satisfaction, and rapidly burned off existing fat.

Results were remarkable, usually within two weeks. Moreover, people reported the "Prozac effect" in great numbers. As psychiatrist Peter Kramer told us in *Listening to Prozac*,

> There has always been the occasional patient who seems remarkably restored by one medicine or anther, but with Prozac I had seen patient after patient become, like Sam, "better than well." Prozac seemed to give social confidence to the habitually timid, to make the sensitive brash, to lend the introvert the social skills of a salesman. Prozac was transformative for patients in the way an inspirational minister or high-pressure group therapy can be—it made them want to talk about their experience. And what my patients generally said was that they had learned something about themselves from Prozac. Like Sam, they believed Prozac revealed what in them was biologically determined and what was merely (experience being "mere" compared to cellular physiology) experiential.[6]

So Slimline gave its customers far more profound benefits than merely no longer feeling fat. In case after case multiplied millions of times, a whole personality changed. On Slimline people not only felt no need to eat, they felt empowered. Many reported that for the first time in their lives, they felt truly free and alive. "Something's changed in my brain," one reported but speaking for thousands, "and I never want to go back."

With both SmartKid and Slimline, there was a remarkable lack of those adverse reactions known euphemistically in medicine as "side effects." Genetic screens and tests allowed versions of these drugs to be almost individually designed to match the peculiar genetic variations of each class of individuals, maximizing the effectiveness of the drug and minimizing side effects.

Of course, such biological changes always have unforeseen effects. A new generation of serotonin re-uptake inhibitors, especially ProzacPlus, has made psychotherapy a dying field. What psychiatrists didn't foresee (and they were the ones in the first few years who really pushed the new drugs), was that nonpsychiatric physicians would soon prescribe the drugs, quickly forcing many psychiatrists out of work. Optical enhancements given to fetuses have been vigorously opposed by optometrists and ophthalmologists, who see them as threats to their livelihoods. A new genetic dental kit for newborns, given to seven-week embryos and carried on an artificial chromosome, has been opposed by the American Dental Association as "unethical" (the dentists claim it would be "eugenic" to have a whole society of children with perfect teeth).

And all this is just the beginning. In 2010, we stand on the brink of many exciting new kinds of genetic therapies for existing disease, of presymptomatic testing for late-onset genetic disease, of genetic screening of sperm, eggs, embryos, and fetuses, of "genetic drugs" individualized to particular patients, and even of possible, permanent cures for genetic diseases through germ-line genetic therapy. If only we are allowed to go forward.

INEGALITARIAN

To the surprise of egalitarians, who had opposed them, use of such drugs actually reduced inequality of certain sorts. People who already had good memories had some improvements with SmartKid, but those with poor memories gained dramatically. Similarly, those naturally thin got no benefit at all from Slimline because it gave fat people a key metabolic gene that thin people already had. Fat people, of course, gained immeasurably, not in weight, but in health and self-esteem.

Of course, some die-hard academics (especially the Canadian Post-Modernist school and the Mary Dalyites) screamed that SmartKid and Slimline were fitting everyone into a bland Procrustean bed. Fortunately, their cries went unheeded. But egalitarianism dies hard, and a pincer movement of the political Left and the political Right kept raising the specter of eugenics. In our own time, *Mother Jones* devotes at least one issue per year to "genetic injustice" and Jeremy Rifkin Jr. has produced three books denouncing the same.

They all rail against the fact that a small percentage of families screen their fetuses for genetic disease, correct any problems in utero, and add enhancements, giving their children a huge biological advantage, and thus, later social and economic advantages.

The fear of biologically based inequality has been one of the most substantial and pervasive objections to genetic enhancement (and also to human cloning). As Robert Wright wrote in 1999 in *Time*: "Sooner or later [if parental choice about genetic disease and enhancement expands] as the most glaring genetic liabilities drift toward the bottom of the socioeconomic scale, we will see a biological stratification vivid enough to mock American values."[7] This was certainly overstated. We think "American values" include personal choice by parents about the number and kinds of children born to a family. Does Mr. Wright deny that such values also include letting families choose the goals of children's development? He implies that taking away choice is more consistent with American values, but perhaps he was just writing sensationally for effect.

There are two entirely different issues here: First, is the new thing in genetic medicine a real human good? Second, if it is, how should it (if at all) be subsidized and made available? The first question is about benefit to humans; the second is one of distributive justice.

We are having a lot of difficulty with opponents who claim that unless we have a way of answering the second question, we should not create goods covered by the first. They say that, in particular, medicine shouldn't be in the business of making people more unequal and, if it's about to, it should cease and desist until we become equal.

As we saw in debates about money for organ donation or assisted reproduction, egalitarians want medical policies to equalize nonmedical aspects of life. Of course, they have tried to ban SmartKid and Slimline. They want to make the clock run backward, making medicine focus only on curing age-old diseases or on rehabilitating victims of accidents.

They always think we don't see their point. "It's bad enough," they complain, "that some kids must go to lousy public schools when others go to elite, private schools. Now inequality will not just be in differing educational environments, but in our flesh and bones. With the new germ-line enhancements, inequality is being permanently etched in our genes. That is unjust."

We do see their point. They want to make everyone equal, and *then* change. We are pessimistic about achieving such social equality and reluctant not to progress. True equality is difficult, perhaps impossible, to achieve, especially if equality is richly defined to include social, economic, and biologically equal prospects in life. As Robert Nozick taught us, if society could somehow wave a magic wand and start everyone equal in the above regards, it would not stay equal long.[8] People will make uneven trades, some will seek certain goals (fame, money) more intensely than others, and some families will sacrifice more for their children than others. All these activities will disturb the initial, equal homeostasis. Magnified millions of times, the instability will be much greater, and one can appreciate how true equality, even if obtained for a brief time, would be impossible to maintain without despotic control over family effort, trades, and individual initiative.

Moreover, when our critics say that genetic enhancements should not be offered until a minimal social equality is achieved, there is another important problem to be addressed. One of the major ways middle-class parents become poor is by losing a job because of the long-term illness of a child, and many of the severe illnesses of children are genetically caused. What realistic hope do poor families have of living middle-class lives when they have children afflicted with long-term genetic diseases? Even if state and federal governments, along with local charities, pay for most of the medical treatment, the family must often provide the at-home, daily care. There is only so much social restructuring that can be done to redress the ongoing inequality that results when some families undeservedly suffer such conditions.

Empirically, we accept that some children cannot be genetically enhanced without inadvertently widening the gap between the high and the low. What we can do, however, is to recognize and plan for this problem. Such planning in part accounted for passage of the National Medical Act of 2008, guaranteeing every U.S. citizen a right to medical care by universalizing Medicare. Thank God this finally came about.

CONCEPTS OF GENETIC DISEASE AND ENHANCEMENT

Many of the old still claim that it's permissible to eradicate genetic disability but not to enhance natural endowments. They argue that genetic screening and therapy deal with disease, whereas enhancement does not.

As history has shown, such an argument falsely assumed a simplistic, factual, biology-only view of disease and health. Our concept of disease is determined partly by our assumptions about normality and abnormality. Moreover, there is no purely factual concept of disease, because our concept is determined partly by underlying evaluative premises.[9] Disease is not just "read off" from facts in nature but is partly an evaluative judgment about whether a particular, often abnormal, characteristic is bad. Extreme strength is statistically abnormal, but not a disease, whereas extreme lack of strength is dysfunctional. Being overweight and myopic is probably statistically normal now in the U.S. population. Gay men and lesbians, about 2 percent of the population, were once considered by the *Diagnostic and Statistical Manual* of the American Psychiatric Association to have a psychiatric disease, but modern evaluative judgments consider that view prejudicial. Masturbation and a desire by women to have sexual relations were once considered evidence of psychopathology.

The concept of disease may be seen as a core with expanding circles around it. As movement proceeds to the outer circles, what is included as a disease becomes more and more controversial. A myocardial infarction is a paradigm of disease; premenstrual syndrome is not. Congestive heart failure is a classic disease; mitral valve prolapse is not.

In genetics, there is always a range of values in any population, and in the evaluative judgments associated with that range, there is always a danger in classifying a merely atypical value as "diseased," for example, homosexuality. One of the reasons why choice about genetics must be a bedrock principle is that what some people regard as a liability (homosexuality) may be regarded by others (gay men and lesbians) as an asset.

Similarly, there was a continuum in phenotypic qualities between correcting genetic disease and attempting genetic enhancement, and doing one always shaded into the other. This continuum could be diagrammed like this:

Disease/dysfunction   Normal functioning   Ideal functioning

In this diagram, the goal of genetic therapy is to go from left to right, to get a patient out of the disease/dysfunction state and to the normal state. Similarly, genetic enhancement is envisioned as going from middle to right, moving a normal person to an enhanced state.

This distinction between genetic therapy and genetic enhancement assumes that the places on the above continuum are fixed, but that assumption turns out to be false: the continuum itself moves forward (to the right). In ancient Greek times, the average life expectancy was only thirty-five years. Wars, plagues, bad water, poor nutrition, lack of antibiotics, and death in childhood contributed to early death. A hundred years ago, the average expected life span of an American was only fifty-six, but for a similar child born in 1999, it was eighty-nine, and now in 2010 (for children advantaged at birth by enhancements), life span is predicted to be 109 years.

Moreover, a remarkable change occurred about the *quality* of the extra years. In the nineteenth century, people aged sixty-five to eighty-five often had uncontrolled diabetes leading to blindness and amputations, crippling arthritis, and exhausting heart disease. Increasingly today, young people expect *at least* a hundred years of high-quality life, which is claimed by some as a new medical right.

In short, the definition of health as ideal functioning changed over time to:

Dysfunction   Normal   Old Ideal   New Ideal

No doubt your ideal of good health is far beyond ours in 2010. Perhaps your ideal is unimaginable to us.

This has not been an easy fight. Our critics insist that the treatment/enhancement distinction must be obtained because: (1) it defines the proper goals of medicine (treatment, not enhancement), (2) it defines the minimum of medical services owed to all people in a just, democratic society (treatment of disease and dysfunction, not improvement), and (3) it prevents eccentrics from thinking the job of medicine is to make a Master Race.[10] To us, the first point simply begs the question by defining *proper medicine* that way. As for the second objection, this distinction is just one way to distribute medical services, and it has the disadvantage of pretending that an evaluative decision is somehow "read off" from biology. We do not think the distinction can bear this weight, for example, most preventive medical services such as vaccines, clean water, and antiseptic surgery are improvements, not simply treatments for medical problems.

What the third objection has in mind is that if enhancement is considered even *possibly* a proper goal of medicine, eccentrics will take this out of normal contexts. From permitting a few couples to enhance children, eccentrics will soon argue that couples are *obligated* to do so and that society should encourage or enforce such obligations. To this our speaker has replied that no sound public policy was ever made that attempted to preclude what eccentrics might or might not do. Eccentrics will do as eccentrics do. In the end, it is evidence, reason, and compassion that sway people.

As another example of the problems of this distinction, consider the controversy in the year 2000 about giving a growth hormone to very young children who were shorter than most in their age cohort. Originally, the idea was that pediatricians would give such hormones to kids who were dwarfish or extremely short, but not to make normal children taller. When all was said and done, it turned out to be impossible to distinguish good from bad uses.

Consider SmartKid and a family of people of average intelligence, where the average I.Q. was 100, and that has a kid who tests at 85 at age six. Here was a paradigm of Smartkid's potential. But consider also another family where I.Q. 135 was the norm, and that had a child who tested at I.Q. 100 at year six. Both families request SmartKid from their pediatrician. Is the first family "good," the second, "bad"?

Many people thought it awful that a family would regard being mentally average as bad. Such people hoped that society would be more accepting of average people or that the family would instill in mentally average kids strong self-esteem. And some such changes did occur.

But the families who chose SmartKid quietly went about their business. Some gave interviews pointing out that some people still criticized infertile couples who often endured many cycles of in vitro fertilization and who paid huge amounts of money for low chances of having a baby. Both kinds of families quietly responded that such personal decisions about having kids and raising kids have traditionally been left up to parents, who were trying to do their best.

More generally, for almost any drug or gene therapy, the line between correction and enhancement has been fluid. Whether it is SmartKid, Viagra, improved muscles for athletic performance (first given to the puny), or Slimline, it is hard to see how a medical treatment can only be given to correct a deficiency, not to add to the norm, especially when the norm covers wide variations.

The above arguments deal in *content*, but *process* arguments make them stronger. In medical contexts, if a real distinction is to be maintained between good and bad uses of a new technique, the physician has to be the commissar. She has to reject the requests of the "bad" patients and only honor those of the "good." Her rejection puts her in the position of not merely judging right and wrong, but judging between different theories of the good life. The latter, of course, is a much more personal and subjective area than is our common morality (where at least we can agree most of the time about what harms people). Physicians are neither inclined nor trained to make such judgments, nor is it in their financial interest to do so. So they do not.

Moreover, once a medicine or drug is approved by the FDA, physicians can use it for any purpose. What, then, is to prevent "normal" patients coming to a physician who wants to pay herself for a genetic therapy officially approved for (and thus, officially reimbursed for) only corrective efforts? Because of this problem, some critics want to go so far in enforcing the corrective/enhancement distinction as to make it *illegal* for a physician to so prescribe a genetic treatment.[11]

When a few states did so, it became a legal nightmare. They had to specify in statutes when correcting low I.Q., short stature, or weak muscle mass ceased to be corrective and began to enhance. State statutes said unwieldy things such as, "Physicians may not medicate a child to be more than 20 percent taller, stronger, or brighter than the child's age-adjusted norm." Certainly that judgment depended on the particular facts of the patient, and even of time and place. In the infamous case of Baby Leo, judges and district attorneys made fools of themselves by prosecuting a physician and parents who had in fact made Baby Leo at age two more than 50 percent taller and smarter than the norm for American two-year-olds (the D.A. even calculated that Baby Leo giggled 50 percent more than normal, using his own two-year-old as a control). Critics thought this was explained because Baby Leo was laughing at the D.A.; others understood why the D.A.'s kid didn't laugh much. In this case, the jury took five minutes to acquit, and no one has been prosecuted since.

Paradoxically, those against any expanded genetic choice for parents agree in one aspect with our arguments. For we argue, in what might be called "hard-won ascent," that there is no logical place to draw the line and to say, "Change up to here but no more." We recognize that our reverse-slippery-slope argument is a double-edged sword that cuts for and against expanded choice. For if there is no logical place to stop until we get to allowing genotypes originated from germ-line changes or human cloning, critics will resist expanded genetic choice in the first place.

Nevertheless, even in our time, it's clear to us that it is not "if" parental choice in genetics will expand but "when." Of course, the "when" might be delayed a hundred years, as often happens in the history of medicine, but we hope, perhaps overoptimistically, that humans will actually base their views on reason and evidence, not on knee-jerk emotion.

MORE CRITICISMS

Our critics also pressed on us with other objections. First, aren't enhancements such as SmartKid self-defeating?[12] No, we respond, because SmartKid doesn't make smart kids much smarter, but really helps mentally challenged kids. Moreover, we shouldn't assume that the point of enhancements is to give some a competitive advantage; instead, it is to make humans better so they can enjoy life more. Teaching kids to play sports, to read, and to play a musical instrument should be valued in just this way: not as ways of obtaining competitive advantage over others, but as expanded ways of enjoying life.

Another objection by our critics is that genetic enhancements are improperly obtained.[13] It is one thing for a person to obtain tranquility through years of hard work in psychotherapy or at weight-loss clinics; it is not the same good to obtain these by taking a pill. Part of the value of these goods, critics say, is in the work of getting there. In short, the "means" matter in how a person gets to a good end, and some means are improper ones that medicine should not embrace.

To this "evil means" argument, we reply: let traditionalists avoid such drugs. We do not want to take away their choice to climb the hard road. Let us realize, however, that not everyone in life is blessed with the resources or the desire to do so. Maybe we do not appreciate the much longer life we live simply because we've always had clean water, and undoubtedly we would appreciate clean water more if we experienced diseases borne by bad water or had to clean and boil our own. Be that as it may, having the good of clean water merely allows most people to seek other, better, higher goods.

Finally, there is the vague objection that anything obtained medically is "inauthentic."[14] Here the idea is that the only true human goods are obtained by effort, will, and thinking. Self-fulfillment comes from success in long-range plans over a lifetime, not by taking genetic medicines.

Again, this position has been conclusively falsified by the people who take Slimline and Prozac. Contrary to this objection, such people uniformly report that they have *only* found their true selves on these drugs. Now they regard their former selves as living in an "inauthentic" fog. As John Stuart Mill taught us, the competent judge is the one who has experienced both states.

Eugenics

Even today, freelance writers and academics pushing their books imply that genetic choice of parents will result in Nazi-control of reproduction. Politicians similarly use *eugenics* as a hot-button phrase to inflame voters and to simultaneously divert them from thinking about real issues such as road repair, containment of suburban sprawl, and funding of better schools.

This is also true with *genetic engineering* and *cloning*. These words carry such powerful emotive associations that they instantly stop thought in most people. Wise people cease to use them because they indicate a paranoid, fatalistic mind-set.

Even by 2000, democratic society had successfully transcended many controversies in reproductive ethics without itself being destroyed. It had assimilated artificial insemination by donor, anesthesia in childbirth (contra the famous passage in Genesis), legalization of abortion, the misguided eugenics movement in the early twentieth century, fears about misuse of amniocentesis, fears about recombinant DNA escaping as "Andromeda Strains," fears about "test-tube babies," fears about misuse of genetic screening, fears about misuse of somatic cell genetic therapy, fears about embryonic research on "tiny human babies" conceptualized as homunculi, false scares that humans had been cloned when only embryos had been twinned or when it was a hoax, and fears about genetic therapy to create a master race.

None of these fears ever materialized in Western democracies. After about 1975, they were always unlikely. Indeed, many powerful institutions checked government against misguided eugenics. Without enumerating all of them, they included a woman's right to abort any fetus up to viability; the Americans with Disabilities Act; the many physicians, professors, journalists, and parents who were disability advocates; sanctity-of-life advocates who wouldn't allow even anencephalic babies to die; and finally, the incredible media coverage by CNN, competing news programs, and talk shows of any controversial issue involving birth and parenthood.

Indeed, at the time we urged those who feared eugenics to carefully study the four-decade-old history of "Baby Doe" cases. These were infants who were born with severe disabilities and whose parents sometimes elected not to pursue aggressive treatment for them with the aim of letting them die. After thirty years of publicity, it became much more difficult for parents to allow such babies to die.[15] Once a baby was born, the United States drastically restricted parental choice. This hardly qualified as eugenics.

Allowing Choice Allows Prejudiced Decisions

One of the objections that arose from thoughtful people went like this: "The dominant culture creates a certain image of an ideal woman and an ideal man through advertising, mass media, and Hollywood movies. Suppose then the qualities pictured in these images just happen to be genetically based. Go further. Suppose you could actually get them all in one package as a genotype that parents could choose. Do we really want a society that allows people to choose their children according to such media-driven paradigms?"

"Moreover," this line of objection continues, "if some parents start originating genotypes of children by cloning and choose the ancestors of such genotypes by trying to come as close as possible to the media-defined, ideal images of men and women, won't that put further pressure on those who are plain and average? Will that be good for children who are disabled?"

This is the fear that Mr. and Mrs. Average American are secretly Nazis. The Master Race will come, not "externally" through dictatorship and state coercion, but "internally" and individually, through the collective decisions of millions of American families, each making their own eugenic decisions about desired qualities in children.

Notice first that this is a *fear*, not a fact. A half-century of science fiction, movies, and political grandstanding have caused that fear. But is it true? By 2010, close to *half* of the children born in the United States were non-Caucasian and Hispanic, black, Asian-American, and of other ethnic origins. Almost all these parents wanted a "child of our own," that is to say, one with genetic ties to them, and almost none choose to gestate an embryo of Caucasian ancestors.

Second, if critics question a pattern of choice that seems too much to follow a suspicious norm, then we can revert to the original, Rawlsian position. As the speaker always asks, "What would the people there choose?" She insists that those who would deny choices to parents today must answer to her.

Third, if some disturbing pattern of choice does emerge that is really bad for people, and agreed to be so by most people, such as female feticide after sonogram in India and China, then these harms can be curbed by regulation (the Chinese can allow a second, female child, if families otherwise were allowed only one). But it is important to respond to real, proven, existing abuses, not imagined ones.

Next, notice the problem of saying in advance what are the approved choices and the forbidden ones. In ethics, there is the Theory of the Right and the Theory of the Good; the former concerns morality; the latter concerns ideals of personal life. We have to largely agree in practice about morality or society can't function, but we don't have to agree about a theory of the good. Whether life is lived best with children or without, married or single, in Montana or New York City, as a vegetarian or meat eater, with or without symphonic music, are matters of individual decision and taste, not common morality.

The only place where some parental decisions about children could be banned in advance is where people clearly agree that such decisions harm children. But that terrain is difficult to find. Do women who divorce their husbands and become lesbians "harm" their children by raising them under "mama 1" and "mama 2" rather than under "mom" and "dad"? How good is the government in finding such terrain? In advance?

Of course, fears about eugenics are wildly speculative, and we thought it irrational to base public policy on them (just as it would have been to base public policy about AIDS on initial fears about this disease). To make public policy this way—to argue that we shouldn't allow a small number of couples to seek better children because it might have indirect, negative effects on some existing average—would be like arguing against a cure for half of the people with spinal cord injuries, because doing so might make the other, uncured half feel worse.

At bottom, the worry here about eugenics stems from a combination of two views, one about how malleable human nature is and one about how unmalleable it is. On one hand, there is the sense that ordinary people are easily manipulated by powerful forces in the media and that existing ideals of male and female beauty are mere cultural artifacts. On the other hand, there is the sense that human nature is basically dark and evil. So when a few parents choose to have better and better babies, people will become better and better, and because of their "dark" nature, will despise the plain and ugly.

Obviously, when contradictory views about human nature are assumed, both cannot be true, and there is something wrong with views based on combining both assumptions. Perhaps a better answer is that evidence has been accumulating that most people easily distinguish between what is true in the movies and what is true in ordinary life. Just because movies and television portray certain phenotypes as ideal, does not mean that ordinary people agree with such judgments, or cannot critically evaluate such images when choosing traits of their own children.

Finally, we are optimists: we see no reason to assume the worst in people, especially about parents in relation to their own kids. Eugenics-from-parental-choice is a widespread fear—the "perfect baby" fear—but it is largely just that, a fear, not an empirical fact.

CONCLUSION

So we hope that you now have a sense of the battles we faced in trying to give humans more choices about genetics and babies. We hope that nothing has gone wrong and even more so, that humans did not go backward and block those who wanted more choices.

Our guess about the future is this: a small number of families use in vitro fertilization and embryo testing at both ends of the spectrum, to prevent horrific diseases in their families or to create the best possible children. Because of the costs, effort, and inefficiency of in vitro fertilization, 99 percent of couples who could use these options do not. As a result, changes in the human genome are tiny: at one end, reducing the number of people with terrible diseases and at the other, enhancing the genomes of some families over many generations. We suspect that among these families, there is great consciousness of genes and intensive education from birth, with all kinds of interesting results, mostly good. All of this, of course, we hope is entirely voluntary and that the government has taken a hands-off policy.

As for somatic, genetic therapies and enhancements that affect existing people and that can't be passed on to a new generation, we predict that Smartkid, Slimline, and other such developments have increased the happiness of many people who would otherwise have been miserable. We predict that many people will reject embryonic testing and somatic enhancements, preferring to be "naturals," and we predict that their choices will be respected.

Finally, we hope that, in reading this letter, you look back on our struggle for acceptance of choice for the few and see it like our struggle a century ago for acceptance of the germ theory of disease—as a battle long-won.

Sincerely yours,

Your Ancestors of 2010

NOTES

1. John Rawls, *A Theory of Justice* (Cambridge, Mass.: Harvard University Press, 1971), 108.

2. "Teen Dies Undergoing Experimental Gene Therapy," *Washington Post*, 29 September 1999, A1.

3. Nicholas Wade, "Of Smart Mice and an Even Smarter Man," *New York Times*, 9 September 1999, A1; Joseph Z. Tsien, "Genetic Enhancement of Learning and Memory in Mice," *Nature*, 2 September 1999, www.nature.com.

4. Vivienne Nathanson, *The Daily Mail* (London), 2 September 1999; quoted in *BioNews*, 9 September 1999. To receive this emailed newsletter, send a message to BioNews@lists.progress.org.uk.

5. Steven Rose, "Mice Given Extra Genes Become Smarter," *The Guardian* (London), 2 September 1999.

6. Peter Kramer, *Listening to Prozac* (New York: Viking-Penguin, 1993), xv.

7. Robert Wright, "Who Gets the Good Genes?" *Time* (11 January 1999): 67.

8. Robert Nozick, *Anarchy, State, and Utopia* (Cambridge, Mass.: Harvard University Press, 1974).

9. H. T. Engelhardt, "The Concepts of Health and Disease," in *Evaluation and Explanation in the Biomedical Sciences*, ed. H. T. Engelhardt and S. F. Spicker (Dordrecht: Reidel, 1975,) 125–41; K. W. M Fulford, *Moral Theory and Medical Practice* (New York: Cambridge University Press, 1989); George Agich, "Disease and Value: A Rejection of the Value-Neutrality Thesis," *Theoretical Medicine* 4, (1983): 27–41; W. M. Brown, "On Defining Disease," *Journal of Medicine and Philosophy* 10, (1985): 311–28.

10. Erik Parens, "Is Better Always Good? The Enhancement Project," *Hastings Center Report*, Special Supplement (January-February 1998): S1–4.

11. This has been called the "schmocter problem," i.e., even if we prevent most physicians from prescribing a new drug, how do we prevent a subclass from doing so who practice "schmedicine." See Parens, "Is Better Always Good?" S6.

12. Ibid., S8.

13. Ibid., S7.

14. Ibid., S11.

15. See Gregory E. Pence, "Letting Impaired Newborns Die," *Classic Cases in Medical Ethics*, 3rd edition (New York: McGraw-Hill, 2000), 196–222.

RE-CREATING OUR GENES:
CLONING HUMANS

If we examine our own experience, we find that most mothers and fathers give absolute and unqualified love to the children they raise, no matter what reasons were or were not considered in their conception, and no matter where or how this conception occurred.

—Lee Silver, *Remaking Eden: Cloning and Beyond in a Brave New World*

Human cloning is not a subject that has seen much reasonable discussion. By now the word *cloning* has so many bad associations from science fiction and political demagoguery that there is no longer any good reason to continue to use it. A more neutral phrase, meaning the same thing, is *somatic cell genetic transfer* (SCGT), which refers to the process by which the genotype of an adult, differentiated cell can be used to create a new human embryo by transferring the genes in its nucleus to an enucleated human egg. The resulting embryo can then be gestated to create a baby who will be a delayed twin of its genetic ancestor.

PARALLELS WITH IN VITRO
FERTILIZATION: REPEATING HISTORY?

As we have seen in previous chapters, any time a new method of human reproduction comes along, critics try to prevent its adoption by citing possible harm to children. The implicit premise: before it is allowed, any new method must prove that only healthy children will be created. Without such proof, the new method amounts to "unconsented-to" experimentation on the unborn. So argued the late conservative, Christian bioethicist Paul Ramsey in the early 1970s about in vitro fertilization (IVF).[1]

Of course, not even sexual reproduction guarantees healthy children every time. Nor can a person consent until he is born. Nor can he really consent until he is old enough to understand consent. The requirement of "consent to be born" is silly.

Jeremy Rifkin, another critic of IVF in the early 1970s, seemed to demand that new forms of human reproduction be risk-free.[2] Twenty years later, Rifkin predictably bolted out the gate to condemn human cloning, demanding its worldwide ban, with penalties for transgressions as severe as those for rape and murder: "It's a horrendous crime to make a Xerox of someone," he declared ominously. "You're putting a human into a genetic straitjacket. For the first time, we've taken the principles of industrial design—quality control, predictability—and applied them to a human being.[3]

Philosopher Daniel Callahan, who founded the Hastings Center for research in medical ethics, argued in 1978 that the first case of IVF was "probably unethical" because there was no possible guarantee that Louise Brown would be normal.[4] Callahan added that many medical breakthroughs are unethical because we cannot know (using the philosopher's strong sense of the word *know*) that the first patient will not be harmed. Two decades later, he implied that human cloning would also be unethical: "We live in a culture that likes science and technology very much. If someone wants something, and the rest of us can't prove they are going to do devastating harm, they are going to do it."[5] (Callahan will be discussed in the next chapter when I discuss whether we should accept natural limits.)

Leon Kass, a social conservative and biochemist-turned-bioethicst, argued strenuously in 1971 that babies created by artificial fertilization might be deformed: "It doesn't matter how many times the baby is tested while in the mother's womb," he averred, "they will never be certain the baby won't be born without defect."[6] In 1997, he predictably was one of the first to condemn human cloning, not as unsafe, but as harmful to the identity of children created.[7]

But no reasonable approach to living avoids all risks. Nothing in life is risk free, including having children. Even if babies are born healthy, they do not always turn out as hoped. Taking such chances is part of becoming a parent.

Without taking reasonable risks, there is no progress, no advance. Without taking such risks, pioneers don't cross prairies, astronauts don't walk on the moon, and Freedom Riders don't take buses to integrate the South. The past critics of assisted reproduction demonstrated a psychologically normal but nevertheless unreasonable tendency to magnify the risk of a harmful but unlikely result. Such a result—even if very bad—still represents a very small risk. A baby born with a lethal genetic disease is an extremely bad but unlikely result. We shouldn't try to avoid all risks. Just unreasonable ones.

HUMANITY WILL NOT BE HARMED

Human SCGT is even newer and stranger sounding than in vitro fertilization. All that means is that it will take longer to get used to. Scaremongers have predicted terrible harm will come to children who are conceived as a result of SCGT, but in fact very little will change. Why is that?

First, to create a child by SCGT, a couple must use IVF, which is an expensive process, costing about $8 thousand per attempt. Most U.S. states do not require insurance companies to cover IVF, so IVF is mostly a cash-and-carry operation. Second, most IVF attempts are unsuccessful. The chances of any couple taking home a baby is quite low—only about 15 percent.

Only about fifty thousand IVF babies have been born in the United States since the early 1980s. Suppose fifty thousand such babies are born over the next decade. How many of these fifty thousand couples would want to originate a child by SCGT? Very few—at most, perhaps, a few hundred.

These figures are important because they tamp down many fears. As things now stand, originating humans by SCGT will never be a common practice. Neither evolution nor the old-fashioned human sex act is in any way threatened, nor is the family or human society. Most fears about human cloning stem from ignorance.

Similar fears linking cloning to dictatorship or to the subjugation of women are equally ignorant. There are no artificial wombs (predictions, yes; realities, no—otherwise we could save premature babies born before twenty weeks). A healthy woman must agree to gestate any SCGT baby, and such a woman will retain her right to abort. Women's rights to abortion are checks on evil uses of any new reproductive technology.

NEW THINGS MAKE US FEAR HARMS IRRATIONALLY

SCGT isn't really so new or different. Consider some cases on a continuum. In the first case, the human embryo naturally splits in the process of twinning and produces two genetically identical twins. Mothers have been conceiving and gestating human twins for all of human history. Call the children who result from this process Rebecca and Susan.

In the second case a technique is used where a human embryo is deliberately twinned in order to create more embryos for implantation in a woman who has been infertile with her mate. Instead of it happening because of a random quirk in the uterus, now a physician and an infertile couple use a tiny electric current to split the embryo. Two identical embryos are created. All embryos are implanted and, as sometimes happens, rather than no embryo implanting successfully or only one, both embryos implant. Again, Rebecca and Susan are born.

In the third case, one of the twinned embryos is frozen (Susan), along with other embryos from the couple, and the other twinned embryo is implanted. In this case, although several embryos were implanted, only the one destined to be Rebecca is successful. Again, Rebecca is born.

Two years pass, and the couple desires another child. Some of their frozen embryos are thawed and implanted into the mother. The couple knows that one of the implanted embryos is the twin of Rebecca. In this second round of reproductive assistance, the embryo destined to be Susan successfully implants and a twin is born. Now Susan and Rebecca exist as twins, but born two years apart. Susan is the delayed twin of Rebecca. (Rumors abound that such births have already occurred in American infertility clinics.)

Suppose now that the "embryo that could become Susan" was twinned, and the "non-Susan" embryo is frozen. The rest of the details are then the same as the last scenario, but now two more years pass and the previously frozen embryo is now implanted, gestated, and born. Susan and Rebecca now have another identical sister, Samantha. They would be identical triplets, born two and four years apart. In contrast to SCGT, where the mother's contribution of mitochondrial genes introduces small variations in nearly identical genotypes, these embryos would have identical genomes.

Next, suppose that the embryo that could have been Rebecca miscarried and never became a child. The twinned embryo that could become Susan still exists. So the parents implant this embryo and Susan is born. Query to National Bioethics Advisory Commission: have the parents done something illegal? A child has been born who was originated by reproducing an embryo with a unique genotype. Remember, the embryo-that-could-become Rebecca existed first. So Susan only exists as a "clone" of the nonexistent Rebecca.

Now, as bioethicist Leroy Walters emphasizes, let us consider an even thornier but more probable scenario.[8] Suppose we took the embryo-that-could-become Susan and transferred its nucleus to an enucleated egg of Susan's mother. Call the person who will emerge from this embryo, "Suzette," because she is like Susan but different, because of her new mitochondrial DNA. Although the "Susan" embryo was created sexually, Suzette's origins are through somatic cell nuclear transfer. It is not clear that this process is illegal. The National Bioethics Advisory Commission (NBAC) report avoids taking a stand on this kind of case.[9]

Now compare all the above cases to originating Susan asexually by SCGT from the genotype of the adult Rebecca. Susan would again have a nearly identical genome with Rebecca (identical except for mitochondrial DNA contributed by the gestating woman). Here we have nearly identical female genotypes, separated in time, created by choice. But how is this so different from choosing to have a delayed twin child? Originating a child by SCGT is not a breakthrough in kind but a matter of degree along a continuum involving twins and a special kind of reproductive choice.

COMPARING THE HARMS OF HUMAN REPRODUCTION

The questions of multiple copies of one genome and its special issues of harm are ones that will not be discussed in this text, but one asymmetry in our moral intuitions should be noticed.

The increasing use of fertility drugs has expanded many times the number of humans born who are twins, triplets, quadruplets, quintuplets, sextuplets, and even (in November 1997 to the McCaugheys of Iowa), septuplets. If an entire country can rejoice about seven humans who are gestated in the same womb, raised by the same parents, and simultaneously created randomly from the same two sets of chromosomes, why should the same country fear deliberately originating copies of the same genome, either at once or over time (two of the McCaughey babies now have long-term problems, one with cerebral palsy, the other has been on a feeding-tube for over a year)?

People exaggerate the fears of the unknown and downplay the very real dangers of the familiar. In a very important sense, riding in a car each day is far more dangerous to children than the new form of human reproduction under discussion here. More than forty thousand people in the United States are killed every year in automobile wrecks, yet few people consider not driving.

In SCGT, there are possible dangers of telomere shortening, inheritance of environmental effects on adult cells passed to embryonic cells, as well as other possible, though currently unknown, dangers. Mammalian animal studies must determine if such dangers are likely to occur in human SCGT origination. Once such studies indicate that there are no special dangers of SCGT, the crucial question will arise: How safe must we expect human SCGT to be before we allow it?

In answering this question, it is very important to ask about the baseline of comparison. How safe is ordinary, human sexual reproduction? How safe is assisted reproduction? Who or what counts as a subject of a safety calculation about SCGT?

At least 40 percent of human embryos fail to implant in normal sexual reproduction.[10] Although this fact is not widely known, it is important because some discussions tend to assume that every human embryo becomes a human baby unless some extraordinary event occurs, such as abortion. But this is not true. Nature seems to have a genetic filter, such that malformed embryos do not implant. About 50 percent of the rejected embryos are chromosomally abnormal, meaning that if they were somehow brought to term, the resulting children would likely be abnormal.

A widely reported but misleading aspect of Ian Wilmut's work was that it took 277 embryos to produce one live lamb. In fact, Wilmut started with 277 eggs, fused nuclei with them to create embryos, and then reduced the results to the best thirteen embryos, which were allowed to gestate further. He had three lambs almost live, with one true success, Dolly. Subsequent work may bring the efficiency rate to 25 percent. When the calves "Charlie" and "George" were born in 1998, four live-born calves were created from an initial batch of only fifty embryos.[11]

Wilmut's embryo-to-birth ratio only seems inefficient or unsafe because the real inefficiency rate of accepted forms of human assisted reproduction is so little known. In in vitro fertilization, a woman is given drugs to stimulate superovulation so that physicians can remove as many eggs from her as possible. At each cycle of attempted in vitro fertilization, three or four embryos are implanted. Most couples make several attempts, so as many as nine to twelve embryos are involved in the process for each couple. As noted, only about 15–20 percent of couples undergoing such attempts ever take home a baby.

Consider what these numbers mean when writ large. Take a hundred couples attempting assisted reproduction, each undergoing (on average) three attempts. Suppose there are unusually good results and that 20 percent of these couples eventually take home a baby. Because more than one embryo may implant, assume that among these twenty couples, half have nonidentical twins. But what is the efficiency rate here? Assuming a low number of three embryos implanted each time for the three hundred attempts, it will take nine hundred embryos to produce thirty babies, for an efficiency rate of one in thirty.

Nor does all the loss of human potential occur at the embryonic stage. Unfortunately, some of these pregnancies will end in miscarriages of fetuses, some well along in the second trimester.

Nevertheless, such loss of embryos and fetuses is almost universally accepted as morally permissible. Why is that? Because the infertile parents are trying to conceive their own children, because everyone thinks that is a good motive, and because few people object to the loss of embryos and fetuses *in this context of trying to conceive babies*. Seen in this light, what Wilmut did, starting out with a large number of embryos to get one successful lamb at birth, is not so novel or different than what now occurs in human assisted reproduction.

Of course, no one wants to subject naive, overly eager or desperate women to late-term miscarriages. More work needs to be done on nonhuman primates before we try human cloning, and when we do try, it's important that the first cases come out healthy (or else everyone will overreact and ban SCGT).

SUBJECTS AND NONSUBJECTS OF HARM

One premise that seems to figure in discussions of the safety of SCGT and other forms of assisted reproduction is that loss of human embryos morally matters. That premise needs to be questioned.

As the previous discussion shows, loss of human embryos is a normal part of human conception and, without this process, humanity might suffer much more genetic disease. This process essentially involves the loss of human embryos as part of the natural state of things. For every human baby successfully born, there seems to be at least one human embryo lost along the way.

In vitro fertilization is widely accepted as a great success in modern medicine. As said, more than fifty thousand American babies have been born this way. But calculations indicate that as many as a million human embryos may have been used in creating such successes.

Researchers often create and store embryos for subsequent cycles of implantation, only to learn that a pregnancy has been achieved and that the stored embryos are no longer needed. Thousands of such embryos can be stored indefinitely in liquid nitrogen. No one feels any great urgency about them, and, indeed, many couples decline to pay fees to preserve their embryos.

These considerations point to the obvious philosophical point that embryos are not persons with rights to life. Like an acorn, their value is all potential, little actual. Faced with a choice between paying a thousand dollars to keep two thousand embryos alive for a year in storage, or paying for an operation to keep a family pet alive for another year, few people will choose to pay for the embryos. How people actually act says much about their real values.

Thus, an embryo cannot be harmed by being brought into existence and then being taken out of existence. An embryo is generally considered such until nine weeks after conception, when it is called a fetus (when it is born, it is called a baby). Embryos are not sentient and cannot experience pain. They are thus not the kind of subjects that can be harmed or benefited.

As such, whether it takes one embryo or a hundred to create a human baby does not matter morally. It may matter aesthetically, financially, emotionally, or in time spent trying to reproduce, but it does not matter morally. As such, new forms of human reproduction such as IVF and SCGT that involve significant loss of embryos cannot be morally criticized on this ground. As such, the de facto ban on research on human embryos by all funding agencies of the U.S. government should be immediately lifted so that important research (stimulated in part by Wilmut's discovery) about cancer and genetics can go forward using human embryos.

STANDARDS OF HARM

Animal tests have not yet shown that SCGT is safe enough to try in humans, and as was pointed out previously, extensive animal testing should be done over the next few years. This means that before we attempt SCGT in humans, we will need to be able to routinely produce healthy offspring by SCGT in lambs, cattle, and, especially, nonhuman primates. After this testing is done, the time will come when a crucial question must be answered: How safe must human SCGT be before it is allowed? This is probably the most important, practical question before us now.

Should we have a very high standard, such that we take virtually no risk with an SCGT child? Daniel Callahan and Paul Ramsey, past critics of IVF, implied that unless a healthy baby could be guaranteed the first time, it was unethical to try to produce babies in a new way. At the other extreme, a low standard would allow great risks.

What is the appropriate standard? How high should be the bar over which scientists must be made to jump before they are allowed to attempt to originate an SCGT child? In my opinion, Callahan and Ramsey's standard is too high. In reality, only God can meet that Olympian standard. It is also too high for those physicians trying to help infertile couples. If this high standard had been imposed on these people in the past, no form of assisted reproduction—including in vitro fertilization—would ever have been allowed.

On the other end of the scale, one could look at the very worst conditions for human gestation, where mothers are drug-dependent during pregnancy or exposed to dangerous chemicals. Such worst-case scenarios include parents with a 50 percent chance of passing on a lethal genetic disease. The lowest standard of harm allows human reproduction even if there is such a high risk of harm (*harm* in the sense that the child would likely have a subnormal future). One could argue that since society allows such mothers and couples to reproduce sexually, it could do no worse by allowing a child to be originated by SCGT.

I believe that the low standard is inappropriate to use with human SCGT. There is no reason to use the very worst conditions under which society now tolerates humans being born as our standard of reference. If the best we can do by SCGT is to produce children as good as those born with fetal-maternal alcohol syndrome, we shouldn't originate children this way.

Between these standards, there is the normal range of risk that is accepted by ordinary people in sexual reproduction. Human SCGT should be allowed when the predicted risk from animal studies falls within this range. *Ordinary people* refers to those who are neither alcoholic nor dependent on an illegal drug and where neither member of the couple knowingly passes on a high risk for a serious genetic disease.

This standard seems reasonable. It does not require a guarantee of a perfect baby, but it also rejects the "anything goes" view. For example, if the rate of serious deformities in normal human reproduction is 1 percent, and if the rate of chimpanzee SCGT reproduction were brought down to this rate, and if there were no reason to think that SCGT in human primates would be any higher, it should be permissible to attempt human SCGT.

PSYCHOLOGICAL HARM TO THE CHILD

Psychological harm is often claimed to be caused by erroneous parental expectations. In particular, there is a widespread belief that any child originated by SCGT would be harmed by unrealistic expectations created by his parents in comparing his future with the life of his genetic ancestor. Call this the argument from parental expectations.

One version of this argument claims that what is wrong about SCGT origination is that it is wrong for a parent "to want a copy of himself." Call this the wrongness of self-replication objection. This popular objection is vulnerable on two points. First, the objection is not about SCGT but about having the wrong motives for creating children. The implied bad motives are those of vanity or narcissism. Some people may claim that it is wrong to have such motives in creating any child, not just for creating a child by SCGT. In any case, the criticism is not unique to SCGT.

Perhaps those who make this kind of objection think that the only kind of child who would be created would be from the genome of one of the parents. But if this were the real problem, then the objector should have no problem if the parent chose the genome of someone else, say a favored uncle or a brilliant aunt. Of course, the worry rarely goes away if this alternative is suggested, allowing us to infer that the real objection here has to do with the novelty of SCGT or something else.

The second problem with the objection concerning self-replication is that it is based on a falsehood. It may be helpful at this point to explain two key terms. The *genome* of an individual is the complete set of his genes. How a genome is expressed in a particular individual is his *phenotype*, the result of the interaction of the genome with the environment. A phenotype is the resulting, entire physical, biochemical and physiological makeup of the individual. Exposing the same genome to different environments creates different phenotypes, for example, where one fetus receives inadequate nutrition during gestation and another superior nutrition.

The idea that the phenotype of a girl originated by SCGT would copy the phenotype of her genetic (nuclear) ancestor is false, and false in myriad ways. Even in the most extreme example, we know that so-called identical twins have tiny differences in their genomes—caused partly, probably, by how much of the X chromosome is inactivated in fetal development, a random process in each twin. Such differences, writ large twenty years later, may account for why even conjoined twins, such as the famous Eng and Chang, may have opposed personalities, to the extent of one being alcoholic and the other a teetotaler.

We also know that the gestational mother of an SCGT-originated fetus will contribute a small number of genes to the resulting child, meaning that the final genome of the resulting child will differ slightly from that of the genetic ancestor. Even at its most basic level, the SCGT child's genome will never be an exact copy of her ancestor's.

Beyond the genome, the new child will have a different environment than her ancestor did, in not just the obvious ways of place and years of upbringing, specific parents, schools, and friends, but in less obvious ways like what the gestational mother does or does not drink, does or does not take, like folic acid and vitamin B supplements, and how much she talks to the newborn during the first two years of her life (resulting, some think, in how many neural pathways for language are formed). So the SCGT child would be neither a genetic nor a phenotypic copy of the genetic ancestor.

Nevertheless, some people who want to originate an SCGT child this way believe they will get a copy of themselves. This raises a new, but much more general question: How important should such false beliefs be in making public policy about bioethics?

This question arose in the 1980s when many people had false beliefs about HIV infection. Some believed that HIV-infected children could infect healthy children at school; some orderlies and hospital aides left food outside the rooms of patients with AIDS, fearing infection if they entered; other fears concerned contamination from public rest rooms, mosquitoes, communion cups, and coins.

Looking back, it was a mistake and wrong to base public policy on such false beliefs. Doing so made irrational fears seem legitimate. The best way to deal with falsehoods is to act as if they are false, while simultaneously educating people about the truth.

Similarly, and with false expectations about SCGT children, prospective parents would need to be educated about what to realistically expect. In this regard, there will be an important role for counselors in clinics specializing in this kind of assisted reproduction. Compare such counselors to genetic counselors, who often see clients who are at risk for a dominant, autosomal genetic disease—such as Huntington's disease—clients who have roughly a 50–50 chance of having the gene. When such clients come to be tested, often their real hope is to discover that they do *not* have the gene. Yet the hopes of such clients must, unfortunately, be disappointed in approximately half the cases.

An important job of the genetic counselor is thus to make such at-risk clients understand (and, perhaps, feel) what they will experience in the event they get an unexpected (or undesired) result. When such counseling succeeds, people no longer have false beliefs and many don't get tested. Such successful counseling explains a recent report in the news expressing surprise that more Americans with such diseases haven't been tested. But this is not really a surprise, given the lack of treatment for many genetic diseases and the possible discrimination by U.S. insurance companies should records indicating a patient has such a genetic disease be created.

One important fact is that SCGT origination cannot be performed outside assisted reproduction clinics. There is a bottleneck and a social check in this particular kind of human reproduction that is not possible for most human sexual reproduction. Thus there is an opportunity to mandate counseling and to make sure that most parents do not have false beliefs about prospective SCGT children. Therefore, because it is generally a bad idea to make public policy based on falsehoods, and because there is a practical way to correct false expectations of prospective parents, this objection to SCGT origination is not a good one.

The objection about the wrongness of self-replication has so far been countered by saying that expectations about self-replication are generally false. But let us now consider a form of this objection that purports to be based not on false expectations but on true ones.

Some people at this point will object, "Yes, it is true that the child would not be an *exact* genetic copy, and yes, the expression as an adult would vary a lot, but still, there will be a lot of similarity between the genetic ancestor and the child. And to that extent, the parental expectations will be based on truth. But it would be wrong to create a child this way because, to the extent that the child is similar to one who has lived before, the parent will have expectations about him that could become true, and again, it is wrong to create children based on such expectations."

This objection against SCGT origination can be called the argument for an open future. Because someone with this genome has lived before, and because this child was created in part (or even mainly) because of the characteristics of this particular genome, the future of the first SCGT-originated child is claimed to be closed in a way not true for every other human child who has ever been born.

This objection can be countered in a variety of ways. First, a comment needs to be made about the general picture of child creation that this objection presents, which is ultimately Kantian in its assumption that a child should be valued in it-self, not as a means to the satisfaction of someone else's desires. As such, a child should be wanted in itself, not for the particular characteristics it might have. What is wrong about SCGT is that every child should have a completely open, com-pletely indeterminate future, shaped not at all by his parent's expectations.

In reply, it can be argued that this sets up a false ideal, not only of why peo-ple have children but also of how they ought to have them. This passive ideal might stem first from historical times, when people had no control over the traits of their children, and second, from a very recent trend to place children on an altar, on which the lives of parents are often sacrificed in order to provide the children with myriad developmental activities, such as computer camps, special schools, and sports.

And is a forced choice really necessary? Isn't this another simplistic dilemma? Why can't I value such a kid both for himself *and* for his similarity to me?[12]

Important as these points are, I want to turn the focus to those things that are considered to be objectionable about parental expectations about SCGT. Now let's assume that parents have been counseled and that, based on primate studies of SCGT, they have good evidence that a child with 99 percent of Woody Allen's or Elle MacPherson's genomes will be more likely than normal to be intelligent or beautiful, respectively. Suppose also that intelligence and beauty are, respectively, what is valued.

One thing that might be considered objectionable is to give parents any choice at all about such characteristics. Many people seem to have such beliefs. The ob-jection here is of two kinds: that such choice is intrinsically wrong or that such choice is indirectly wrong because it will create undesirable consequences.

People who believe that choosing characteristics is intrinsically wrong often believe that it is up to God, nature, or evolution to determine who is born and with what characteristics and that it is wrong for humans to make such choices.

People who make this objection often get confused at this point between ob-jecting that: (1) human society should not make choices about which human characteristics are desirable and try to bring about babies with such characteristics, or (2) particular parents should not make choices about which human characteristics are desirable and try to bring about babies with such characteristics. The first is associated with eugenics and dictatorial states taking away reproductive choice from couples; the second is an expansion of current reproductive choice for couples. Fears and concerns about the first are not arguments for curtailing choice in the latter, but the opposite, for a strong and regularly exercised right to reproduce as one chooses is a good check against reproductive coercion.

Most people don't really believe (2) that choosing characteristics in future people is wrong. People send their children to one school rather than another based on such beliefs. Prospective parents use genetic tests to test embryos and fetuses to avoid severe genetic disease and abort those that test positive. Mothers avoid cigarettes and alcohol during pregnancy to optimize the environment of their fetuses.

To argue that such choices are wrong ultimately is to accept reproductive fatalism. Such fatalism must also apply to who gets pregnant, and it is not surprising that those who oppose genetic choice also usually oppose abortion and contraception. The Vatican at least is consistent.

In the Vatican's consistency, there is an insight. On its view, humans should accept everything that happens as God's will and attempt to change nothing. Each pregnancy or disease is as it should be, and God has a sufficient reason for it. To oppose His will is sinful pride.

To link up to a previous topic, once we let people choose to take contraception or to abort because they don't want to be pregnant, it is hard to justify not letting them abort because a fetus has a genetic disease, because it will be deaf, or because it will be a dwarf. Once we allow for abortion to avoid dwarfism or deafness, it is hard not to allow medical treatments at birth designed to overcome dwarfism, such as doses of human growth hormone, or to overcome deafness, such as cochlear implants. Implicit in these decisions is the judgment that being short or deaf is undesirable and being tall or able to hear is good. Once those judgments have been made and it becomes possible to choose children who are able to hear better or be taller, it becomes difficult to say why it is wrong to allow parents to make these kinds of choices. (Indeed, once this is granted and once it becomes possible to do so, it becomes difficult to say why parents should not be able to permanently modify their germ cells to create taller or nondeaf children, but that is another topic.)

Here it will be objected that some parents will put too much weight on one characteristic, such as intelligence or the current ideal of female beauty, and then be very disappointed when the child does not measure up. Put more generally, to emphasize a connection between the value of the child to the parents and the particular characteristics the child might have—characteristics that are uncontrollable, unpredictable, and morally arbitrary—is to harm any child who lacks the desired characteristics or who does not possess them to the degree desired by the parents.

If a parent has an obsession about one characteristic (for example, the high I.Q. of a famous ancestor) and believes that an SCGT-originated child will certainly have that characteristic, then what we have is a variation on the first objection. It is very likely false that the child will have a particular characteristic to the same degree that the famous ancestor did. Moreover, it will often be a particular combination of traits that is desirable, not just a trait such as physique or skill in solving mathematical puzzles, and such a combination will very likely be the result of the child's environment and education.

A variation of this argument concerns parents who focus on looks in planning for an SCGT-originated child. In the famous Baby M case of commercial surrogacy in the United States, the Sterns chose the surrogate mother, Mary Beth Whitehead, only because she had a physique that looked like Mrs. Stern. In this, we all know now that they were very ill informed, for they disregarded the importance of personality, intelligence, and perhaps, mental illness, in making their selection. Similarly, couples seeking embryos or eggs for implantation in older infertile women in the United States often choose mainly on the basis of the looks of the genetic ancestors. That, of course, is a simpleminded way to choose.

The real truth of modern genetics is that everything is complex. There may be no simple genetic test for breast cancer, because there may be hundreds of variations, so that to tell a woman she has no genetic risk would first require testing for each and every variation. In the context of cloning, the author of the scientific section of the NBAC's *Cloning Human Beings* summarized:

> Indeed, the great lesson of modern molecular genetics is the profound complexity of both gene-gene interactions and gene-environment interactions in the determination of whether a specific trait or characteristic is expressed . . . recent scientific findings have revealed that a "one-gene-one-disease" approach is far too simplistic. Even in the relatively small list of genes currently associated with a specific disease, knowing the complete DNA sequence of the gene does not allow a scientist to predict if a given person will get the disease.[13]

And if a disease can't be predicted, how much more difficult will it be to predict traits such as wit or dexterity? Many qualities of the phenotype will be multifactorial at the genomic level and multifactorial at the level of gene-environment interaction, such that how any quality gets created in a phenotype will be hard to foresee. Originating children by cloning will not deprive them of an open future as much as people think.

But learning that will be a matter of education and experience. People will need counseling. Personally, I have great faith in prospective parents and what they are capable of learning. Their learning curve here will be short: a few well-publicized cases of silly parental expectations will teach thousands, if not millions, about the lessons of Genetics 101.

We are also somewhat hypocritical to pick on cloning when it comes to parental expectations. Over the past decade, thousands of American couples have adopted abandoned Chinese babies. Some of these babies—most female—are identified in their adoption papers by the milepost number they were found near, as in "Milepost baby #1324." Many of these adoptive couples say that they feel very good about adopting these abandoned babies. One theme repeated by many of these parents is that they expect that the child as an adult will be grateful to the parents for having adopted them. "After all," one parent told me, "without us, she would have died." These adoptive parents have very strong expectations that their adoptive child will feel grateful and see them in good, if not morally heroic, terms.

From a Kantian view, these expectations are not in the best interests of the child. No parent should expect his or her children to see him or her as a saint. It is far better for everyone involved if adoptive parents merely expect their child to see them as any other child sees any other parent. According to the Kantian ideal, children fare best if no special expectations are put on them.

Nevertheless, no one criticizes such parents for these expectations, and no one is suggesting that, because of such expectations, adoption of Chinese babies should be made illegal. Because people understand adoption and the recent need to turn to China for babies (because of a lack of healthy American babies), no one wants to ban this practice. Why, then, do people want to make human cloning illegal based on similar kinds of "bad" expectations?

CONCLUSIONS

To the extent that the argument from parental expectations is based on false beliefs, it can be countered first by saying that we should not make public policy on false beliefs and second, that social mechanisms are available to counter any damage done by these false parental beliefs to SCGT-created children. Even then, some small damage from expectations might occur, but if so, it is likely to be no greater than damage caused by any other failed kind of parental expectation about children created by traditional sexual means.

On the other hand, even if SCGT-created children correctly fulfill parental expectations, for example, the SCGT-originated child from Woody Allen's genome really is witty, this does not negate the free will of such children to lead other kinds of lives. An adult created from Woody's genes might decide to live in Phoenix running a plumbing business, being an outdoorsman, and not being regarded by his friends as funny or even comical.

In such matters, it is best not to take an a priori position, as so many did in the past when condemning various forms of assisted reproduction, which later proved benign. Critics claimed that amniocentesis would allow parents to choose only perfect children and to abort any child who was not. What critics missed is that by the time a fetus has been gestated for six months, almost all parents really want to keep it and would choose to abort it only *when forced to choose against a terrible genetic disease, not against having a child.*[14] Similarly, critics claimed that in vitro fertilization would be abused, in combination with embryo transfer, and would allow parents to create only perfect babies. Again, such critics underestimated how much such procedures cost as well as the fact that most infertile couples are content to get *any baby at all* in a process where only 15 percent of such couples actually take home a baby.

If twenty years of experience with new forms of assisted reproduction have taught us anything, it is that we should be open-minded about new techniques of human reproduction and skeptical about claims of monstrous babies and about great harm to society and that we should think better of most parents than to caricaturize them as selfish.[15]

Most of the arguments against human cloning, whereby an existing person's set of genes would be re-created, are bad ones. Whether they focus on physical or psychological harm, the arguments appeal more to fear than to fact or logic. In this they resemble other arguments against ethical change in medicine that we have considered previously in this book.

NOTES

1. Paul Ramsey, *Fabricated Man: The Ethics of Genetic Control* (New Haven, Conn.: Yale University Press, 1970).

2. "What are the psychological implications of growing up as a specimen, sheltered not by a warm womb but by steel and glass, belonging to no one but the lab technician who joined together sperm and egg? In a world already populated with people with identity crises, what's the personal identity of a test-tube baby?" J. Rifkin and T. Howard, *Who Shall Play God?* (New York: Dell, 1977), 15.

3. Rifkin quoted in Ehsan Masood, "Cloning Technique 'Reveals Legal Loophole,'" *Nature* 38, Internet site, 27 February 1987.

4. "Was Louise Brown's Birth Ethical?" *New York Times*, 27 July 1978, A16.

5. Knight-Ridder newspapers, 10 March 1997.

6. Leon Kass, "The New Biology: What Price Relieving Man's Estate?" *Journal of the American Medical Association* 174, no. 19 (November 1971): 779–88.

7. Leon Kass, "The Wisdom of Repugnance," *New Republic* 2 (June 1997): 5–12.

8. Leroy Walters, "Biomedical Ethics and Their Role in Mammalian Cloning," Conference on Mammalian Cloning: Implications for Science and Society, 27 June 1997, Crystal City, Virginia.

9. National Bioethics Advisory Commission (NBAC), *Cloning Human Beings: Report and Recommendations of the National Bioethics Advisory Commission* (Rockville, Md.: U.S. Government Printing Office, 1997).

10. A. Wilcox et al., "Incidence of Early Loss of Pregnancy," *New England Journal of Medicine* 319, no. 4 (28 July 1988): 189–94. See also J. Grudzinskas and A. Nysenbaum, "Failure of Human Pregnancy after Implantation," *Annals of New York Academy of Sciences* 442 (1985): 39–44; J. Muller et al., "Fetal Loss after Implantation," *Lancet* 2, (1980): 554–6.

11. Rick Weiss, "Genetically Engineered Calves Cloned," *Washington Post*, 21 January 1998, A3.

12. I owe this point to Kelly Smith.

13. National Bioethics Advisory Commission, "The Science and Application of Cloning," *Cloning Human Beings* (Rockville, Md.: U.S. Government Printing Office), 32–3.

14. I believe I learned this point, and this way of putting it, from John Fletcher, who often stresses it.

15. I am indebted to Rosamond Rhodes and Kelly Smith for comments on an earlier version of this chapter. Part of this chapter originally appeared in the *American Philosophical Association Newsletter* (Philosophy and Medicine) 98, no. 1 (Fall 1998): 104–6 (copyright Gregory Pence).

7

RE-CREATING NATURE: PATENTING HUMAN GENES?

That as we enjoy great Advantages from the inventions of others, we should be glad of an opportunity to serve others by any invention of ours, and this we should do freely and generously.

—Benjamin Franklin, display in atrium, Franklin Museum of Natural History and Science, Philadelpha, Pennsylvania

Recently, a chorus of Cassandras has told us that terrible things will happen because human genes are now subject to the protection of patents. Scientists who work for pharmaceutical companies assert just the opposite, claiming that without such protection, new "genetic medicines" will not be developed.

What is the truth? Are such patents the worst thing that has happened to medicine since Columbus started to exploit the West, or do patents promise smarter people, healthier kids, and cures for age-old diseases?

By a series of flukes, the United States has not experienced the public debates that have wracked England and Europe about patents on plants, animals, and human genes. The U.S. Supreme Court and U.S. Patent and Trademark Office (PTO) have granted legal patent protection to discoverers of sequences of human DNA. Because of these decisions, Americans have not had the intense national debate that, for example, Icelanders had before they voted in a national election to allow the Swiss-based Novartis to study their national gene pool, to patent any useful genes found there, and to develop any genes useful as medicines.[1]

Because there has not been public discussion, there is currently little public understanding of these issues. This chapter discusses them and attempts to shed a little light on this continuing controversy.

PATENTING "LIFE"?

In 1980 in a famous decision, *Diamond v. Chakrabarty*, the United States Supreme Court awarded patent protection to geneticist Ananda Chakrabarty for his creation of a genetically modified organism designed to clean up oil spills.[2] In doing so, the Court set a precedent, declaring that organisms that are alive can receive the protection of patents if they have been altered or genetically modified.

Previously, U.S. patent law did not generally allow patents on "products of nature" or on "nature's handiwork," that is, naturally occurring things such as rocks, plants, and chemical elements (although it did allow patents on new, large complex molecules). As analyst and philosopher Claudia Mills observed in 1985, the Supreme Court ruled that Chakrabarty's discovery was "not nature's handiwork, but his own . . . the relevant distinction [is] between products of nature, whether living or not, and human-made inventions."[3] This Court agreed that, because Chakrabarty had changed the genes of an organism to make it clean up oil, it was a "human-made invention," not something occurring wild in nature.

Chakrabarty was a narrow ruling based on the Court's interpretation of Congress's intent in drafting particular legal bills. However, in the similar *In re Bergy* case in 1981, a lower court quite explicitly emphasized that "the fact that microorganisms . . . are alive is a distinction without legal significance."[4]

Chakrabarty and *In re Bergy* have been discussed in public mainly by critics such as popular writers Jeremy Rifkin and Ted Howard, biologist/bioethicist Leon Kass, Harvard biologist and activist Richard Lewontin, and Indian activist and physicist Vandana Shiva. These critics have largely set the crucial "first step" in this public debate and in doing so, may have led the public to focus on the wrong issues.

Reacting against *Bergy* in 1981, Kass argued that "life" should not be patentable or exploited for profits.[5] To come under the protection of patents, and hence, to be bought and sold, he claimed, degrades humanity. He said it was like allowing medical corporations to patent "mule," that is, to patent the Platonic essence of an animal.

In 1980, Ted Howard wrote an amicus curiae brief for Jeremy Rifkin's People's Business Commission (later known as the Foundation for Economic Trends). It was filed at the Patent Office and opposed patents on human DNA.

Howard argued that such patents would devalue human life and implied that genetically changed life "will have been categorized as less than life, as nothing but common chemicals."[6] Howard complained in 1977 that *Bergy* treated life as "an industrial tool," not as something sacred, and claimed that "life itself, even at its lowliest, is invested with a sanctity that the patent process defiles."[7] Leon Kass similarly saw *Chakrabarty* as symbolizing the triumph of private interests over the common good, the subjugation of science to profit, and the winning of the worldview that sees nature as something to be owned and manipulated.[8]

Until recently, these views were the only ones that became public. However, in the early 1990s, some scientists started to defend patents on human DNA in public, while others criticized such attempts. Before deciding whether any such claims are true, we need to know something about the history of this debate over the past twenty years.

A GENETIC GOLD RUSH?

The approximately 140 thousand genes account for a small part of the three billion base-pairs that compose human DNA, but genes carry the information necessary for cells to produce (they "encode") the proteins that cells generate and utilize in regulating biological functions. A gene is a sequence of DNA of variable length.

Once geneticists and others discover what sequences of DNA compose our genes, it will be up to physiologists to determine, via cellular, animal, and human studies, how these gene-protein interactions find expression in human traits and abilities. This next physiological step will likely take years. After that, researchers in psychology, epidemiology, sociology, and early childhood education will take over in determining how a similar genotype can be expressed differently in different environments to create different phenotypes. While these studies are going on, medical researchers will be attempting to find genetic therapies for inherited diseases caused by lack of protein functions (e.g., cystic fibrosis) or other genetic defects caused by chromosomal complications (e.g., Down's syndrome).

Using enzymes, it is possible to find "tags" for the DNA sequences that help produce the proteins used by cells. These tags are called "expressed sequence tags" (ESTs). An EST is a unique DNA sequence that is part of a gene and that is useful in making gene maps. The sequence of DNA in an EST exists in nature; it is not created. From one important point of view, it is basically information.

Such ESTs can be identified without formulating the entire expression of the full DNA of the sequence. In the early 1990s, controversial entrepreneur Craig Venter pioneered the use of fast, big computers to discover ESTs. The work in discovering ESTs comes in identifying them by synthesizing primers and using a technique called "polymerase chain reaction" or PCR. A list of ESTs provides a template for where genes might be and, more important, where genes might be that have significant medical or biological aspects.

Early in his career, Venter worked for the National Institutes of Health and in 1990 urged it to file for patents on the ESTs that he had made. In 1991, NIH so filed and in doing so, provoked an outcry from scientists in the private sector. These scientists feared that government patents on such DNA fragments would compete with their own patenting efforts. There was also an outcry from scientists in universities, who believed that the NIH's patents would hinder the free and open exchange of ideas that ideally characterizes scientific investigation.

Patents issued on ESTs were thought by critics to be odd because the filer of the patent has no idea what genes the ESTs mark or whether those genes are associated with any disease or trait. Second, and very important, if the ESTs are seen as *information* and not as things, then *copyright* would seem to be the appropriate form of protection of intellectual property, not patents.[9] (But perhaps neither is appropriate because both patent and copyright traditionally cover things that someone invents, not something preexisting in nature.)

Historically, government has funded research and let private researchers reap the profits. For example, the U.S. government has spent many millions developing an artificial heart, but when the time came to bring such hearts to possible profitable use, it let private companies file for patents on specific devices such as the Jarvik-7.[10]

NIH might have continued to do so but for Venter's views and for what had been occurring in U.S. research universities. Although many academic researchers claimed that human DNA sequences should not be patented, this belief was not shared by the provosts and presidents of their institutions. Within the past decade, every major research university has aggressively pursued patent rights on discoveries made by its scientists, so much so that the administrator responsible for leading this effort usually has a very high rank within that university. Whether it is a new stent in cardiology, an oncomouse at Harvard, or a new therapeutic protein, universities see future monies coming to them from acquiring such patents. For example, Columbia University made $96 million in the 1998–99 fiscal year from licensing agreements in biotechnology, and UAB made $10 million.[11]

In 1991 when Venter discovered a way to use high-speed computers to speed up the drudgery of finding and marking genes, it must have seemed to him that everyone but NIH was filing patents on every possible discovery in biotechnology. Hence, having the federal government do so was no more unnatural than, say, the University of Michigan, doing so.

However, because of the outcry (both nationally and internationally), and because the Patent and Trademark Office initially rejected NIH's application, NIH in 1994 withdrew its application. Nevertheless, the whole three-year process created immense controversy and spurred private companies to file their own applications for patents on ESTs and DNA sequences.[12]

What was particularly controversial is that patents on ESTs seemed to cover large batches of human DNA where the researchers had no idea how the proteins regulated the expression of various biological functions or human conditions. In other words, a patent had been granted where the holder of the patent didn't know what the "invention" did. Very odd.

As we shall see in the next section, there were already criticisms about "patenting life" or "owning life" through patents on genes and criticisms about religious symbolism of allowing such patents. Hence it was somewhat extraordinary for patents to be granted in the midst of such ignorance. Writing in *Science* magazine, Leslie Roberts characterized this change as "a land grab, a preemptive strike that would promote a worldwide stampede to garner patents on essentially meaningless pieces of DNA."[13] Roberts and others worried that such changes would result in scientists not cooperating with each other (which has in fact happened to some extent),[14] hoarding their knowledge in hopes of later profits and refusing to cooperate in the worldwide sharing of genetic knowledge that had previously characterized work on the Human Genome Project.

Venter left NIH in 1991 and formed his own nonprofit company, the Institute for Genomic Research ("TIGR"), to discover ESTs, and its for-profit partner, Human Genome Sciences (later called Celera Genomics). The latter was also backed by venture capitalists hoping to profit from drugs and proteins developed from TIGR's knowledge.[15]

Because of Venter's rapid success in finding ESTs, scientists working for universities and government increasingly panicked and asserted that TIGR and similar for-profit companies must be stopped or thwarted. Meanwhile, Venter was upsetting everyone by showing how much faster the job could be done when someone is motivated by profits rather than by government salary or grants, and also (critics said) by "cherry picking" the areas of DNA ripe for genes.

Jeremy Rifkin saw TIGR and other biotechnology companies as evil international corporations, scarfing up the "green gold" of humans by patenting their DNA and genes. Rifkin predicted that patents on human DNA would allow for-profit corporations to control the world medical economy the way OPEC once

did with oil.[16] Harvard biologist and socialist Richard Lewontin similarly criticized such patents as part of a larger critique of medicine and biotechnology:

> Activities that previously were the direct result of human interactions—entertain-
> ment, emotional support, learning, recreation, child care, even human blood and
> transportable organs or the use of the womb—have now entered the marketplace,
> where human relations hide behind impersonal buying and selling. Each time a
> new aspect of life is commoditized, some resistance is expressed as outrage at the
> debasement of previous values.[17]

Lewontin's view shows how opposition to patenting genes can be part of a
larger view that opposes financial incentives for organ transfers and paying for
reproductive help.

All these criticism had their effect. To head off Venter acquiring a monopoly
on ESTs, the Human Genome Project's director Francis Collins announced
that it would speed up its work, and Britain's Welcome Trust announced that it
would kick in several billion dollars to prevent human genes from being privately patented. Furthermore, pharmaceutical giant Merck announced that,
working in conjunction with Washington University in St. Louis, it would make
all its discoveries public by filing them immediately on the Internet (the legal
significance of which will be discussed soon).

Merck's move was the last paradox in the whole debate: where before the
federal government had attempted to patent what (some said) should be a public good, now a for-profit pharmaceutical company was using private money to
give the results of its research to the public. Critics replied that Merck had
nothing to lose in doing so because its commercial strength was in bringing
identified drugs through the complicated maze of human drug trials, not in
using genetic databases to identify new drugs.[18]

One lesson from this brief history is that simplistic characterizations of scientists are misleading, especially the common picture of "pure" scientists
working in universities or working at NIH versus "greedy" scientists working
for biotechnology companies. Given a chance, many universities filed application for human DNA fragments and ESTs discovered by their scientists. Some
scientists have gone back and forth between private corporations and public
institutions. Some academic, biology departments allow their professors to
work for private companies, which pay both the professor and department,
and—even though no peer-reviewed publications result from such activities—
count such activities as the professor's "research." More commonly, many scientists have complicated arrangements whereby they work for both universities and private biotechnology companies, often necessitating complex
conflict-of-interest agreements.

RELIGIOUS CRITICISMS

Some religious leaders criticized the decisions by the U.S. Supreme Court and the U.S. Patent Office to allow patents on human DNA sequences. On May 18, 1995, nearly two hundred of them issued a statement at a press conference in Washington, D.C., entitled, "Joint Appeal against Human and Animal Patenting."

Two years later, in 1997, the Hastings Institute, the famous thirty-year-old think tank located north of New York City and devoted to bioethics, brought together representatives from religion and biotechnology industries to find common ground on the ethics of patenting human DNA.[19] They made no progress, because neither side budged in its view.

At this meeting, attorneys for industry argued that patents were necessary to ensure return on investment by start-up biotechnology companies, that patents had already been issued on identified genes in plants and nonhuman animals, and that some future DNA sequences would be very useful in gene therapy and medicine. For patent attorneys, the idea that patents could be bad was not a concept they were willing to entertain.

Religious leaders retorted that the patent attorneys failed to understand the *symbolism* of a society saying that human DNA and genes could be patented, marketed, and commercialized. The president of the Southern Baptist Convention's Christian Life Commission emphasized that altering or creating new life forms was a "revolt against God's sovereignty and the attempt by humankind to usurp God and be God."[20] He further elaborated that:

> Human beings are pre-owned. We belong to the sovereign Creator. We are, therefore, not to be killed without adequate justification (e.g., in self-defense) nor are we, or our body parts, to be bought and sold in the marketplace. Yet, the patenting of human genetic material attempts to wrest ownership from God and commodifies human biological materials and, potentially, human beings themselves. Admittedly, a single human gene or a cell line is not a human being; but a human gene or cell line is undeniably human and warrants different treatment than all non-human genes or cell lines. The image of God pervades human life in all of its parts. Furthermore, the right to own one part of a human being is *ceteris paribus* the right to own all the parts of a human being. This right must not be transferred from the Creator to the creature.[21]

In this quotation, we again see the connection between opposition to patents on human DNA and opposition to paying people for transplantable organs or other body parts.

At about this time, Jeremy Rifkin and a scientific partner, New York Medical College biology professor Stuart Newman, did a clever thing, designed to be a reductio ad absurdum of the idea of patenting human DNA sequences. They filed for a patent on a human-animal chimera, a biological hybrid composed of 51 percent nonhuman animal DNA and 49 percent human DNA. Of course, they had no such animal in the wings and had no idea of how to create such an animal. Then again, patents were being issued on ESTs for which the holders of the patents had no idea what genes the ESTs contained or what the genes did. The idea here was to force thought about how much of "the human" could be patented.

As it turns out, the U.S. Patent Office cannot legally reject an application for a patent on moral grounds. Partly this is by design to prevent politics from entering the process (e.g., pacifists opposing patents for new weapons). As such, the commissioner of the Patent Office was in a panic about how to reject Rifkin's application on technical, nonmoral grounds, without simultaneously undermining previous decisions of his office. Eventually, this application for a patent was rejected because it was "too human," forcing the Patent Office to acknowledge—according to one specialist in patent law—"the relatively thin legal ice upon which its policies" rest on patenting human DNA.[22]

Sociologists Dorothy Nelkin and M. Susan Lindee believe that many in religion have come to see human DNA and genes as representing "the social and cultural functions of the soul. It is the essential entity—the location of the true self—in the narratives of biological determinism."[23] In the popular culture that has infiltrated religious thought, "Genes 'R Us," reveals the true person and his future. Nelkin and Lindee continue:

> The gene has become a way to talk about the boundaries of personhood, the nature of immortality, and the sacred meaning of life in ways that parallel theological narratives. Just as the Christian soul has provided the archetypal concept through which to understand the persona and the continuity of self, so DNA appears in popular culture as a soul-like entity, a holy and immortal relic, a forbidden territory.[24]

The essential objection by religious leaders was clear: just as human organs should not be sold, so human genes should not be owned. These criticisms raise questions for us: Do patents on human genes confer ownership? And does the symbolic, religious value of genes mean that they should not be made into commodities?

JOHN LOCKE ON THE FRONTIER

Almost three hundred years ago, English political philosopher and physician John Locke described how resources could go from natural, commonly owned things into private property. In his *Two Treatises of Government*, Locke argued that it was in the self-interest of each person to form a government to escape from the state of nature where, as Hobbes later said, life is "solitary, poor, nasty, brutish, and short."

Locke's argument was distinctive in its appeal to property to justify the founding of government. Indeed, the primary goal of government is to protect property and make secure rules as to its transfer and protection. How, then, does what is wild in nature become private property for Locke? His famous solution is worth quoting in full:

> Though the earth, and all inferior creatures be common to all men, yet every man has a "property" in his own "person." This nobody has any right to but himself. The "labour" of his body, and the "work" of his hands, we may say, are properly his. Whatsoever then he removes out of the state that Nature hath provided, and left it in, he hath mixed his Labour with it, and joined to it something that is his own, and thereby makes it his property. It being by him removed from the common state Nature placed it in, hath by this labour something annexed to it, that excludes the common right of other men. For this "labour" being the unquestionable property of the labourer, no man but he can have a right to what that is once joined to, at least where there is enough, and as good left in common for others. (II, 27)

Elsewhere he adds another important insight, "'tis Labour indeed that puts the difference of value on every thing" (II, 40). In sum, and as commentator Peter Laslett concludes, these two statements by Locke "are perhaps the most influential statements he ever made."[25]

Although Locke's justification is famous and underlies the concept of property rights in Western capitalism, not everyone agrees with him. Indian Vandana Shiva is an ecologist, physicist, and grassroots activist for poor farmers against international biotechnology companies. She argues in her book *Biopiracy* that:

> The land titles issued by the pope through European kings and queens were the first patents. The colonizer's freedom was built on slavery and subjugation of the people with the original rights to the land. The violent takeover was rendered "natural" by defining the colonized people as nature, thus denying them their humanity and freedom.
>
> John Locke's treatise on property effectively legitimized this same process of theft and robbery during the enclosure movement in Europe. Locke clearly articulated capitalism's freedom to build as the freedom to steal. Returning private property to the commons is perceived as depriving the owner of capital of freedom. Therefore, peasants and tribespeople who demand the return of their rights and access to resources are regarded as thieves.[26]

Locke goes on to give an example of property in a kind of life, and the questions he asks are very relevant to whether property rights in biology should cover life-forms, processes that create them, or the services of people that maintain and transfer them:

> He that is nourished by the acorns he picked up under an oak, or the apples he gathered from the trees in the wood, has certainly appropriated them to himself. Nobody can deny but the nourishment is his. I ask then, When did they begin to be his? When he digested? Or when he ate? Or when he boiled? Or when he bought them home? Or when he picked them up? And 'tis plain if the first gathering made them not his, nothing else could. That labour put a distinction between them and common. That added something to them more than Nature, the common mother of all, and so they became his private right. (II, 28)

Similarly, the hunter who kills a deer in the commons, or a fisherman who removes a fish from the ocean, makes those animals his property by "mixing his labour" in the taking (II, 30).

However, Locke always makes an important proviso: the nut-gatherer and hunter must not take *all* the nuts or kill *all* the deer, but leave enough behind for the common good of others. Nor would it seem that a person can own more land or property than his "labor" can utilize.

Locke emerges in history as a thinker who wanted to provide a justification for the existing claims of property of the English upper class. He assumes that land and things were owned commonly before government and become private property through "mixing labor" and the laws of government. How applicable Locke's model is to patenting genes will be discussed in the next section.

PROTECTING COMMON HUMAN HERITAGE: VANDANA SHIVA

Locke's model of property assumes that agricultural or industrial development is the proper way for land, or biological products, to be transformed, and indeed, that they *should* be transformed this way. Locke undoubtedly had in mind the vast American frontier and the discovery of new lands. As many have pointed out, his view characteristically ignores the fact that native peoples already existed on those lands and did not regard the land as something that could be parceled into parts and owned privately by individuals.

From the point of view of native peoples, mixing labor with land in Locke's sense (enclosure) does not improve, but spoils, land. Moreover, many critics would agree with native peoples who dispute Locke's assertion that mixing labor allows one to own, not just the crops derived from the land, but the land itself. Indeed, if the land is not used for decades, doesn't Locke's own analysis imply that such land is no longer privately owned?

Vandana Shiva believes that Locke's account is incorrect and immoral. She sees the current patenting of rare genes of indigenous peoples as similar to taking their land: both acts create wealth through the theft of what properly belongs to the original inhabitants: "The creation of property through the piracy of other's wealth remains the same [today] as 500 years ago."[27]

For her, people are already being exploited by drug companies such as Shaman Pharmaceuticals that use the knowledge of native shamans to find new drugs. The same companies are now collecting blood all over the world, hoping to isolate rare, valuable genes and to patent them for their own profits, returning nothing to the original sources and peoples.

In 1492, Queen Isabella and King Ferdinand granted Christopher Columbus the rights of "discovery and conquest," and one year later, Pope Alexander VI declared all lands discovered by Columbus west and south of the Azores to be the property of these same monarchs. Just as papal bulls and charters legitimized the pirating of native peoples, so Shiva thinks that today the General Agreement on Tariffs and Trade (GATT) treaty legitimizes the stealing of the biological resources of native peoples by Western companies. "The vacancy of targeted lands has been replaced by the vacancy of targeted life forms and species manipulated by the new biotechnologies. . . . The freedom that transnational corporations are claiming through intellectual property rights protection in the GATT agreement on Trade Related Intellectual Property Rights (TRIPS) is the freedom that European colonizers have claimed since 1492."[28]

Instead of foreign lands, the "colonies" now sought are biological, from the hidden secrets of a native shaman to the rare, disease-curing genes of indigenous peoples. As Shiva correctly points out, certain potentially valuable "cell lines of the Hagahai of Papua New Guinea and the Guami of Panama are patented by the U.S. Commerce Secretary."[29] She says,

> At the heart of Columbus's "discovery" was the treatment of piracy as a natural right of the colonizer, necessary for the deliverance of the colonized. At the heart of the GATT treaty and its patent laws is the treatment of biopiracy as a natural right of Western corporations, necessary to the "development" of Third World communities. Biopiracy is the Colombian "discovery" 500 years after Columbus. Patents are still the means to protect this piracy of the wealth of non-Western peoples as a right of Western powers.[30]

Shiva thinks the Western idea of owning and patenting forms of DNA is part of a basket of Western evils. These include reductionist science, exclusion of intuition and non-Western ways of knowing, environmental destruction, exploitation of animals, arrogance, and sexism.

One of her interesting critiques lies in exposing certain contradictory stances of biotechnology companies. As we have seen, in applying for patents on plant, animal, and human genes, scientists must prove that something new has been created that does not occur in nature. Take the example of genetically modified food, for example, Bt corn. To patent such corn, a company must argue that what is being patented is something artificial, man-made, and not naturally occurring. On the other hand, when it comes to exporting Bt corn or seed to other countries, the same company claims that there is nothing really new in these plants and animals, and hence, nothing dangerous to the environment or to people. Thus, there is a contradiction in saying (when applying for a patent) that a genetically altered tomato is new and also that the tomato is not new in safety or nutrition compared with traditional tomatoes (in marketing the genetically enhanced food).

It is thus understandable that Europe in 1999 has been so skeptical about allowing imports of U.S. gene-altered plants and food. So far, most European nations have not agreed with the Convention on Biological Diversity, which would have allowed introduction of U.S. gene-enhanced seeds and crops around the world.[31]

Shiva also makes the same point in terms of rights and responsibilities. Owners of the DNA-changed organisms claim the right to own and profit from the changes, but seek to avoid responsibility for any damage caused by such new organisms. Although this is a natural strategy for doing business and maximizing profits, it is philosophically inconsistent. Japanese businesses have a better, more consistent view, as seen when the director of Japan's nuclear industry bowed in apology to neighbors hurt by accidental exposure to radiation in 1999.

PROPERTY RIGHTS

Although it contains some insights, Locke's account of property is simplistic and designed to justify the status quo of his time. In the two hundred years since Locke wrote, U.S. and English common law have analyzed property in much more complex ways. One leading theory today is to see property as consisting of a bundle of *rights*.

Seeing property as a bundle of rights has two points. The most important point is to cast off the old way of seeing property as just a thing. In the old conceptualization, a thing is either owned or not owned, like a switch that is either "on" or "off." The new way conceptualizes property as a bundle of rights, which is to see it not as a thing but as a collection of rights that emphasize the *relationship* of a person to a thing.[32]

Similarly, to say that property is not just one right but a "bundle" of rights is to imply that the rights we have about property are plural and must be analyzed separately. It is to imply that a particular right may be separated or assigned without separating or assigning the other rights.

Such property rights are rarely absolute because others can always be affected by what I do with my property. If I pollute the water, those downstream suffer. If I create and let loose a lethal organism that devours all life in the stream, I hurt others. Courts in England and the United States have struggled for centuries with seeing freshwater rivers as private versus public goods. Railroads in the United States came to be seen as private goods with public uses, and hence, subject to regulation. The U.S. Supreme Court in 1877 in *Munn v. Illinois* even said that grain elevators and public warehouses could fall under legal regulation as businesses involving the public's interests. As philosophy of law scholar Theodore Benditt explains it:

> Though some would reject it, and though there is often great controversy in particular cases, it is fair to say that it is widely believed that the exercise of property rights can have profoundly adverse effects on the well-being of the public, that the welfare of the public cannot be held hostage to private rights, and that at least sometimes property can be required to carry the burden of important public interests—even without compensation.[33]

Not being a thing but a bundle of rights, not being one but many rights (where each may be separable), property has both private and public dimensions. As such, even if patents protect some aspects of property in human DNA, the public may still have legitimate interests in human DNA that must be protected.

WHY WE HAVE PATENTS

The general question of the justification of property has a subsidiary question about the justification of the specific kind of protection of intellectual property rights known as patents (intellectual property also covers trade secrets, copyrights, and trademarks).

Why do we have patent laws in the first place? The two chief reasons for patent law are to: (1) reward the efforts of scientists in discovering useful inventions and (2) to promote the general good. From an economic view, if there were no way to recover costs, why would anyone invest their savings to form capital? The way such inventors are rewarded is by hope of economic gain, and the way humans express their desire for the useful things invented is by buying them.

So strong was the belief that these were good reasons that the founders of the U.S. government put them into the U.S. Constitution. Article I, 8, clause 8 of the U.S. Constitution gives Congress the authority "to promote the Progress of Science and useful Arts" by issuing copyrights and patents.

It is important to note that patent laws do not confer ownership of *private goods* but instead confer rights about *public goods*. Public goods that are intellectual property, such as books, music, or art, are protected by copyright; public goods, such as new drugs, devices, and inventions, are protected by patent law.

One of the most astute commentators on this subject, patent lawyer Pilar Ossorio, observes that such public goods are characterized by the qualities of nonrivalrous competition and nonexcludability.[34] Such public goods differ from personal (or private) property rights because personal property rights give ownership and possession as well as the right to exclude others from use or possession. So my property rights in my house give me the right to own, possess, and use the house and to exclude others from doing the same.

The patent lawyers at the Hastings Center meetings argued, correctly, that patent laws do not give the possessor the right to own the thing patented, that is, to any private property resulting from goods being made from the patent. Patent laws only give the possessor the right to exclude others from "making, using, selling, offering for sale, or importing patented items." Hence, Leon Kass is incorrect and wrong to assert that a patent on a gene gives the possessor of the patent ownership of the gene, and even more globally, incorrect to generalize from one gene to a conglomerate of genes making up the Platonic essence of "mule."

This point bears emphasis. As Ossorio stresses, "Patents do not confer ownership of the thing patented. No particular thing or class of things belongs to a patentee by virtue of her patent. If a person owns a bicycle, then a particular bicycle belongs to her, but if a person has a patent on a bicycle, it is entirely possible that such a person does not own or possess a bicycle."

Thus, rights about patents do not give complete ownership rights, only partial ones. Kass was thinking of property as an all-or-nothing thing, not as a collection of rights. It is also true that just because I have a patent right does not mean I have the other rights commonly associated with a piece of property or idea.

Granting someone a patent on a particular human gene or a DNA segment does not give the holder of the patent ownership of something in all humans with this particular DNA. The holder of the patent would not have the right to extract this DNA out of anyone who had it.

Finally, an important function of patents is to facilitate the spread of new knowledge. Once a patent application is accepted, the information becomes public knowledge. Anyone can go to the U.S. Patent Office and inspect a patent to see how something works. Thus, by giving inventors the right to exclude others from making, using, or selling the invention for twenty years (from the date of filing of the application), the underlying knowledge that led to the invention may also be made public.

WHY PATENTS ON DNA FRAGMENTS ARE VALUABLE

Patents on ESTs or DNA sequences are valuable in different ways. A patent on a DNA segment allows the holder of the patent to sell his right to a company that might use it to develop some medicine, or to develop a diagnostic test for a disease associated with this DNA segment, or to reproduce the DNA segment by various biological processes.

Most products that benefit humans and that develop from new genetic knowledge will emerge from the hard work of late-stage development. As said, such development will be by physiologists and research physicians in developing specific human drugs, blood-clotting factors, growth hormones, agents such as interferon and erythropoietin, and tissue plasminogen activator (TPA), a drug used to mitigate the effects of stroke.[35] So far, holders of patents on DNA sequences have made money by selling the right to use the sequences to other research companies, especially companies that hope to develop such mid-stage products.

One real-world example of such mid-stage development occurred when the biotech company Amgen obtained a patent for a gene sequence that governed creation of the protein erythropoietin, which stimulates production of red blood cells in the body and which is missing in the blood of people in renal failure. Amgen created a genetically engineered version of this protein, Epogen, which is taken by thousands of people on hemodialysis. As a result of this patent and of licensing companies to make this protein, Amgen earns $400 million in annual sales.[36] Another such DNA sequence might regulate and hence be used to develop a diagnostic test for a genetic disease, genetic dysfunction, or desirable genetic trait based on the proteins encoded by these sequences of DNA.

Nevertheless, a patent on a human DNA fragment differs substantially from many late-stage products in medicine, because such a patent is the ground floor of any subsequent building. Whoever controls this ground floor could hold up all tests involving this region of DNA, could hold up manufacture of similar sequences for late-stage products, and could hold up development of innovative therapies.

NATURAL HERITAGE ARGUMENTS

Critics say it is one thing to patent DNA fragments that are commonly available in people in North America. It seems quite another to seek such fragments in ethnic groups around the world whose genes may protect them against common human diseases.

Consider the NIH's interest in 1991 in the Hagahai of Papua, New Guinea, as described in one article in a law review:

> The Hagahai are a 260-member, hunter-horticulturist group which first made contact with government and missionary workers in 1984. The Hagahai are of particular interest to the NIH because tribe members carry the gene that predisposes humans to leukemia, yet they do not manifest symptoms of the illness. The NIH aspires to understand what protects the Hagahai from developing leukemia. Further, the NIH desires to reap the financial benefits of potential pharmaceutical treatments that may be the by-product of their [sic] research.[37]

Some critics believe that international distributive justice requires that if a gene is isolated from the Hagahai that can be used to treat leukemia, the Hagahai should benefit financially. After all, it is their gene that might protect us against leukemia or help us cure it.

Beliefs about the justice of this claim vary considerably. If a DNA segment is seen as just a special case of a drug, then the question arises as to why the Hagahai should profit in a way they would not for any other drug. For example, the anti-organ-rejection drug cyclosporin-A was discovered in fungus brought home by researchers after a vacation in a foreign land, one of thousands of other samples. This particular sample turned out to work, but the costs of proving it, and the costs of finding out that the others did not, were huge.

As Shiva's criticisms illustrate, undeveloped countries resent the "biological piracy" of Western biotechnology companies in raiding their natural resources for valuable human DNA, animal products, and valuable plants. Certainly the U.S. model in treating Native American Indians was shameful. Moreover, just because we have not compensated indigenous peoples in the past does not mean it was right not to do so.

For pharmaceutical companies to send out agents to pry medicinal secrets from native shaman seems sleazy and unjust. In the same way that a physician can use the Internet to maintain the persona of omniscience (and harm patients) or use it to empower patients with joint-decision, so biotechnology companies can simply exploit the natural resources of indigenous peoples or develop joint partnerships that empower them and make them stakeholders in developing successful medicines. Such a strategy encourages long-run cooperation, mutual respect, and sharing of knowledge and seems to be the wisest, most humane, and most just way to do this kind of business.

In other words, it is one thing to patent a common sequence of human DNA; it is another to patent a unique sequence of human DNA peculiar to a certain ethnic group and then to give that group none of the resulting profits. Had they known what they were giving up, would they have consented to this biological mining of their genes? Indeed, how does one prove their *informed* consent in the first place, especially for peoples such as the Hagahai?

PUBLIC OWNERSHIP ARGUMENTS

Perhaps the strongest argument against the permissibility of patents on human DNA is that this very basic stuff of humans should be controlled by all humans as a public good, not privately by individuals or corporations. As John Locke would say, we all own our basic DNA just in being embodied persons, and the only question now is whether government grants someone rights to it without our permission. (Remember that for Locke, land is commonly owned before government legitimizes private property; so our genes are commonly owned before government legitimizes patents over them.)

This argument assumes that it makes sense to say that humans now "own" their DNA. Yet such a notion probably does not make sense. It is unclear how something could be owned when the owner has no idea what it is, where to find it, what to do with it, how to replicate it, test for it, sell it, or do anything at all with it. What ownership rights could be left over?

Then again, one could make the same argument against the very idea of issuing patents on human DNA sequences at a time when the holders of the patent also cannot answer the above-mentioned questions. Moreover, as we've seen, patents don't confer all, or most, of the bundle of rights covered as property.

I think what most people claim, when they think about humans "owning" their DNA or genes, is that such things should not be covered by patent law because such a strategy will not benefit humans. This view asserts that the best way to produce medicinal goods for humans is open, shared knowledge among scientists, a public listing of new genetic discoveries in a public forum such as the Internet, and a lack of secrecy and monopolistic control.

That is, even on the relational, "bundle of rights" view of property and patents, letting one person or company control all the informational relationship of a sequences of DNA may not be in the public's interest. Francis Collins, head of the Human Genome Project, opposes patents on human genes because he believes that such basic research knowledge should not be patented but openly shared. He believes that new genetic tests and drugs will emerge faster with public ownership.

Notice that the above argument, which is implicitly utilitarian, differs in kind from religious arguments that DNA should not be patented because of its negative symbolism or that such bits of "life" should not be patented because they are "preowned" by God. The argument here is about the best means to the ends wanted by all: more knowledge, better drugs, and more ways to prevent genetic disease.

In this argument, few people dispute the claim that biotechnology firms must make money at some point to recoup their capital investments and that they need patent protection of products to do so. U.S. research corporations pursing biotechnology products spend at least half their revenues and capital on research and development, and without the protection of patents, it is hard to see how they could continue to do so. Moreover, such firms have given the United States a lead over biotechnology firms in other countries. The real question then is at what point should such patent protection commence? To answer this question, we need to look at some of the philosophical underpinnings of U.S. patent law.

THE USEFULNESS OF A PATENTABLE THING

We have already mentioned that until recently a patent should not be granted on something occurring naturally in the world but instead needs to be something created or invented. A patent is not supposed to cover the discovery of a new substance, such as a chemical element. So patents do not cover laws of nature, theoretical concepts, or unaltered plants and animals.

How then can DNA segments be patented? They would seem to be just like chemical elements or unaltered plants, namely, something discovered in nature but not altered by man. One answer is from the following 1997 survey in a law journal:

> In determining the patentability of DNA sequences, courts have generally looked to rules which have evolved for chemical inventions. In this context, DNA sequences are considered to be large chemical compounds, and may be patented as compositions of matter under the same principles previously applied to smaller molecules, such as those in many pharmaceuticals. Although patent claims to naturally occurring DNA sequences might be expected to trigger the "products of nature" rule, courts have upheld patent claims covering "purified and isolated" DNA sequences as new compositions of matter resulting from human intervention. Thus, DNA that has been isolated and sequenced in considered patentable subject matter under Patent Statute, and as such product claims may be directed to the DNA sequence of a gene or a portion of a gene, to novel protein products having a specified degree of purity or minimum activity, or to various products containing the DNA sequence.[38]

While it is certainly true that late-stage products of the DNA sequence, such as proteins or diagnostic tests, should be patentable, the question remains whether naturally occurring DNA sequences are not natural "products of nature" and hence, unpatentable by law.

One further test of a successful application for a patent is that it must show that the invention has *concrete usefulness* and is not just a theoretical idea. Simple sequencing of DNA segments (i.e., identification of them) appears to *flatly violate* this requirement of practical utility. Knowledge of such segments is valuable as a research tool, not as a way of making useful products for humans.

Nevertheless, in February 1997, the Patent and Trademark Office decided that such DNA sequences did indeed fulfill the requirement for practical utility because they "were useful for purposes including chromosome mapping, chromosome identification, and tagging genes of known and useful function."[39] Scientists working for NIH and in academia disputed this decision, retorting that such DNA segments were only useful as tools to further basic research.

One other requirement of a successful application for a patent is interesting: the invention must be "nonobvious." If the knowledge contained in the application for the patent is already public, then it is considered "obvious." NIH, Merck, and the Wellcome Trust decided to put each strand of DNA they discovered immediately on the Internet, making each one universal, public, and hence, "obvious." This was a deliberate strategy to undercut the efforts of commercial firms such as TIGR. The more that is publicly identified, the more that is unpatentable.

CONCLUSIONS AND A PROPOSAL

In view of the history of this debate and the arguments on both sides, I believe the U.S. Patent and Trademark Office made a mistake in allowing patents on DNA fragments and ESTs and that continuing to grant such patents is not in the public interest. I think the patents were on things that were in fact "products of nature" and on things that had no foreseeable practical utility. For these reasons, the Wellcome Trust, Merck, and the NIH arm of the Human Genome Project are right to get as much of human DNA as possible into the public domain.

Many of the criticisms of leftist critics such as Rifkin, Shiva, and Lewontin were irrelevant because they targeted every kind of financial incentive in the new biology. Similarly, Kass's early criticisms and religious leaders' later criticisms about life being "owned" through patents were not accurate. Granted, genes symbolize important things about humans, but the issues here are far more complex than came out in public discussions.

Even on John Locke's view, patents on DNA sequences cannot be justified. It would be like giving the first person into the land the right to dam the river and hence, to control all the water necessary to cultivate all the land down-stream, or giving a patent on the mouth of the river, such that no one could land or go upstream without paying a toll. As mentioned, the U.S. Supreme Court struggled mightily with just such conflicting claims about rivers and harbors, trying to balance private and public interests in such "water property."

From the point of the U.S. Constitution, the purpose of patents is to promote "Science and the *useful* Arts." But such promotion is done through specific, *useful* products and inventions, not monopolistic control of the basis for making such future real products and inventions.

In utilitarian terms, patenting DNA sequences is a barrier to the free exchange of ideas about genetics, as many in the academic scientific community have concluded. In this particular case, the eagerness of the PTO and the government to help business, and the biotechnology business in particular, backfired.

Of course, much of this debate from a utilitarian point of view is fine-tuning about the fastest way to create new drugs derived from new knowledge about genetics. Obviously, diagnostic tests for genetic diseases, proteins derived from studying the functions of newly discovered genes, and new drugs derived from the study of genetics should be patentable.

One strategy that holders of patents may employ is refusal to sell licenses for their products to competitors, thus creating a monopoly for their company. Such a strategy has created enormous profits for drug companies that have discovered a particular, valuable drug. However, it would seem foolish for the PTO to allow similar control over ESTs and DNA fragments that are at a very early stage compared with the products that aid humans. This would allow one company to have monopolistic control over whether and how other companies not just develop competing products but do very basic research.

As University of Pennsylvania bioethicist Jon Merz has argued, one compromise is for government to allow patents on human DNA sequences but to require *mandatory licensing* of such patents at a reasonable fee set by the courts or a federal agency.[40] Mandatory (a.k.a. "compulsory") licensing is a legal strategy in which manufacturers holding a patent on a process or drug are not allowed to withhold issuing licenses to other companies to use the same process or make the same product. The holder of the patent must still be paid for use of his patent. However, instead of a commercial negotiation, a government body such as a court or agency sets the royalty for each license.

Mandatory licensing occurred in the fall of 1999 when the government of South Africa passed legislation covering AIDS medicines allowing mandatory licensing and "parallel importing." The latter allows drugs for HIV infection to be sold in South Africa at a much lower price than U.S. drug companies charge in developed countries. The former allows South African companies to manufacture drugs for HIV infection and pay U.S. drug companies some royalties for doing so but exempts such companies from paying whatever the U.S. companies demand. Both of these exemptions are legal under current international trade agreements.[41]

Millions of HIV-infected Africans had no chance of getting life-saving drugs for HIV infection without these two changes. U.S. drug companies opposed the exemptions, and Albert Gore was on their side early in his campaign for president until AIDS activists dogged his speeches so much that he quietly changed.

The strategy of mandatory licensing is especially important in medicine when a company holds a patent on part of a DNA chain, say, for a genetic disease controlled by a larger chunk of that chain, and any diagnostic test for that disease must include the smaller part controlled by the company. Without mandatory licensing, the company can hold up diagnostic testing for the disease or hold out for a very high fee each time a test is done, because a complete test cannot be done without covering the part its patent protects. It is hard to see how allowing a company to hold such tests hostage is in the public interest.

Companies may complain that they need a return on their investment, but they do not need an *outrageous* return, which they might be able to generate if they could block all other genetic tests until other companies paid for the right to use the patent they hold on a particular sequence of DNA. That is, patents on ESTs could create a *government-created* monopoly over diagnostic, presymptomatic genetic tests that is not in the public interest.

The fact that human DNA sequences do not actually create useful products, despite the 1997 ruling by the PTO to the contrary, is a reason to enforce mandatory licensing. The government was on shaky ground in the first place in granting such patents, but it can now minimize the damage by requiring mandatory licensing of all DNA patents.

As I have said repeatedly, it is important to discuss the role of money in medicine and medical research, and this chapter has certainly been preoccupied with such a subject. I have also emphasized in this book that, when talking about money, compromises are usually possible and we should avoid the either-or fallacy of altruistic purity vs. anything-goes commercialism. So to my conclusion:

Patents on human DNA sequences have been granted, and this decision will likely not be overturned (although some high-level federal court could still alter these precedents). Given that we might have to live with this precedent, we should encourage mandatory licensing agreements for holders of patents on human DNA sequences, and by doing so, we can mitigate the bad effects of patents on human DNA while preserving some protection for the scientists who did the original work.

Our discussion of property as a bundle of rights shows how mandatory licensing is compatible with patents on sequences of human DNA. Patents confer some of the rights associated with property, and patents on intellectual property confer some of these rights. In this particular case of sequences of human DNA as intellectual property, we can confer patent protection for private *benefit plus mandatory licensing for public benefit*. Because property is not something one either has totally or does not have at all, this compromise is in accord with modern thinking about the concept of property.

Finally, the symbolic status of human genes also deserves some attention. As Mark Hanson noted, we should avoid each of two extremes: genetic reductionism, when *too much* value is given to genes' relation to personhood, and opposite extreme, which denies *any* value of genes in constructing personhood.[42] Somehow we must find a middle way between these two simplistic extremes.

NOTES

1. Michael Specter, "Decoding Iceland," *New Yorker*, 7 June 1999, 49–62.
2. *Diamond v. Chakrabarty*, 447 U. S. 303 (1980).
3. Claudia Mills, "Patenting Life," *Report from the Center for Philosophy and Public Policy* 5, no. 1 (Winter 1985): 13.
4. Ibid., 13.
5. Leon Kass, "Patenting Life," *Commentary* 72, no. 6 (December 1981): 45–57.
6. Jeremy Rifkin, *The Biotech Century* (New York: Tarcher/Putnam, 1998), 42.
7. Mills, "Patenting Life," 13.
8. Kass, "Patenting Life."
9. This point is owed to Robert Angus of UAB's biology department.
10. Gregory Pence, "Artificial Hearts: Barney Clark," *Classic Cases in Medical Ethics: Accounts of the Cases that Shaped Medical Ethics*, third edition (New York: McGraw-Hill, 2000), 299–320.
11. Carey Goldberg, "Across the U.S., Universities Are Fueling High-Tech Booms," *New York Times*, 8 October 1999, A1.
12. Amy E. Carroll, "A Review of Recent Decisions of the United States Court of Appeals for the Federal Circuit," *American University Law Review* (Summer 1995): 44.
13. Leslie Roberts, "NIH Gene Patents: Round Two," *Science* 255 (1992): note 18, 912.
14. Bernie Wuethrich, "All Rights Reserved," *Science News* 144 (4 September 1993): 154–7. At the October 1999 meeting of the American Society of Bioethics and Humanities, University of Pennsylvania, bioethicist Jon Merz presented results of a study showing that some labs are not offering genetic tests because of difficulty getting licenses on patented genes.
15. Rebecca S. Eisenberg, "Genetics and the Law: The Ethical, Legal, and Social Implications of Genetic Technology and Biomedical Ethics: Intellectual Property at the

Public-Private Divide: The Case of Large-Scale DNA Sequencing," *University of Chicago Law School Roundtable* 3, no. 557 (1996).

16. Jon F. Merz, "Disease Gene Patents: Overcoming Unethical Constraints on Clinical Laboratory Medicine," *Clinical Chemistry* 45, no. 3 (1999): 327.

17. Richard Levins and Richard Lewontin, *The Dialectical Biologist* (Cambridge, Mass.: Harvard University Press, 1985), 199.

18. Eisenberg, "Genetics and the Law."

19. Mark J. Hanson, "Religious Voices in Biotechnology: The Case of Gene Patenting," Special Supplement, *Hastings Center Report* (November-December 1997).

20. Statement by Richard D. Land to the National Press Club, 18 May 1995. Quoted in Hanson, "Religious Voices," 3.

21. Richard D. Land and C. Ben Mitchell, "Patenting Life: No" *First Things* 63 (May 1996): 20–2.

22. Rich Weiss, "U.S. Denies Patent for Part Human, Part Animal," *Washington Post*, 17 June 1999, A6.

23. Dorothy Nelkin and M. Susan Lindee, *The DNA Mystique: The Gene as a Cultural Icon* (New York: W. H. Freeman, 1995), 41–2.

25. Peter Laslett, "Introduction to John Locke's *Two Treatises of Government*," John Locke, *Two Treatises of Government* (New York: Cambridge University Press, 1960), 116ff.

26. Vandana Shiva, "Privacy Through Patents," *Biopiracy: The Plunder of Nature and Knowledge* (Boston, Mass.: South End Press, 1997), 3.

27. Ibid., 2.

28. Ibid.

29. Ibid., 4.

30. Ibid., 5.

31. Rick Weiss and Justin Gillis, "U.S. Lobbies against Biotechnology Trade Limits," *Washington Post*, 13 February 1999; (*Birmingham News*, 14 February).

32. I owe this point to Theodore Benditt. See his *Rights* (Lanham, Md.: Rowman & Littlefield, 1982), 55ff.

33. Theodore Benditt, "Locke: The Individual, the Public, the State," in *Philosophy Then and Now*, ed. N. Scott Arnold, Theodore M. Benditt, and George Graham (Malden, Mass.: Blackwell, 1998), 461.

34. Pilar Ossorio, "Legal and Ethical Issues in Patenting DNA," *A Companion to Genethics: Philosophy and the Genetic Revolution*, ed. Justine Burley and John Harris (New York: Oxford University Press, 2000). I am grateful to her for sharing her essay with me a year before it appeared in print.

35. Courtney J. Miller, "Comment: Patent Law and Human Genomics," *Capital University Law Review* 26, no. 893 (1997), Internet citation.

36. Paul J. Riley, "Comments: Patenting Dr. Venter's Genetic Findings: Is the National Institutes of Health Creating Hurdles or Clearing the Path for Biotechnology's Voyage into the Twenty-First Century?" *Journal of Contemporary Health Law and Policy*, Catholic University of America 10, no. 309 (Spring 1994): note 32.

37. Patricia A. Lacy, "Gene Patenting: Universal Heritage vs. Reward for Human Effort," *Oregon Law Review* (Summer 1998): 77.

38. Courtney J. Miller, "Comment: Patent Law and Human Genomics," *Capital University Law Review* 26, no. 893 (1997), Internet citation.

39. Ibid.

40. Jon F. Merz, "Disease Gene Patents: Overcoming Unethical Constraints on Clinical Laboratory Medicine," *Clinical Chemistry* 45, no. 3 (1999): 327.

41. Mark Weisbrot, "Dollars and Lives: Weak Shame Powerful over AIDS Drugs and Win," *Birmingham News*, 27 September 1999, 9A.

42. Mark Hanson, "Gene Patenting and Commodification," presented 30 October 1999 at the second annual meeting in Philadelphia, Pennsylvania, of the American Society of Bioethics and Humanities.

8

RE-CREATING OURSELVES: NO LIMITS

The technology underlying cell repair systems will allow people to change their bodies in ways that range from the trivial to the amazing to the bizarre. Such changes have few obvious limits. Some people may shed human form as a caterpillar transforms itself to take to the air; others may bring plain humanity to a new perfection. Some people will simply cure their warts, ignore the new butterflies, and go fishing.

—K. Eric Drexler, *Engines of Creation: The Coming Era of Nanotechnology*

In medicine today, many naysayers warn that we must accept natural limits, that we spend too much on medical care, that we are too materialistic, that physicians are being forced to provide futile care, that we are narcissistic in wanting better bodies than we inherited, that we are vain in wanting to live too long, and that all the above show our warped priorities. If we were wise, we would accept our natural limits, not ask medicine for what it cannot deliver, and redirect research dollars to more socially useful ends.

So goes a dominant line of thought in modern medicine and bioethics. It ran through previous chapters, when critics told us to accept needless deaths from lack of organ donors, to accept lack of children rather than to commercialize reproductive help, to ban genetic enhancements, and to fear human cloning. To change the order of things, we are told, is futile, hubris, and unnatural.

But what, exactly, is behind this kind of thinking? For one thing, it is closely connected to discussions about medical futility in medical ethics. On this view, medicine should rehabilitate where it can and cure disease where it can; where it cannot, it should accept natural limits and let life end with dignity.

This attitude in turn is linked to a deeper attitude about medical research. Because medicine should cure and rehabilitate, anything more is frivolous. After a certain point, resources used for improvement ought to be spent on more important social needs, such as education and the environment. There is a fixed pie, such that a big slice for medical research means a smaller slice for other, needy, social goods. In general, we should recognize medical futility in clinical practice, save money, and limit new medical research.

This line of thought also opposes enhancements of the body and mind; such improvements are considered improper. What links this opposition to the former topics is a shared concept of the natural and a corollary that it is wrong to go beyond it. Physicians who do everything possible in futile cases by trying to thwart a natural death harm patients and waste expensive financial resources of society. A society that spends too much on medical research deceives itself that it can one day conquer death and disease. Similarly, when medicine tries not just to cure and heal, but to improve and to enhance, it also violates natural parameters. Such hubris will be punished by failure.

So goes this family of views. These views are also linked by what they propose as the cure. A very widespread view in medicine and bioethics is to say that the solution to all these problems is becoming clear about the *proper goals of medicine*. If we could discover them, then we would know which treatments are futile, which denials of treatment are morally permissible to save money, and which enhancements forbidden.

I shall argue in this chapter that these views are not nearly as plausible as they seem to their champions. Even the idea of medical futility, which has become the new mantra in end-of-life care, is not nearly so objective as it is normally assumed to be. I shall also argue that it is a mistake to follow philosopher Daniel Callahan, who argues that we should limit progress according to the natural, proper goals of medicine. Next, and more philosophically, I will argue that it will be empirically impossible for not only *all* people, but even *most* people, to agree about the proper goals of medicine. Finally, this conclusion has important implications for risk taking by competent adults in the new medicine of the twenty-first century, especially risk taking in pursuit of "improper" goals of medicine.

ETHICAL AND UNETHICAL MEDICAL FUTILITY

A widespread view is that medicine does and should pursue certain proper goals, such as restoring health, curing sickness, and alleviating suffering. All these goals are within the traditional, natural limits of medicine. Nothing fancy or science-fictionish here. It is not the job of medical scientists to challenge those limits or to improve upon Mother Nature.

Physician Lawrence J. Schneiderman and bioethicist Nancy Jecker argue just so in their seminal book on medical futility, *Wrong Medicine: Doctors, Patients, and Futile Treatment.*[1] For them, what makes medicine "wrong" is trespassing beyond natural limits of life and the body.

Schneiderman and Jecker mainly stalk futile medical interventions at the end of life, where there comes a time in every life where further medical action is pointless. When a terminal disease has won, it is appropriate to be fatalistic. Further attempts to combat it produce only pain and misery. Stoical acceptance is then appropriate. This is the time for palliative care and hospice. It is then that those attacking medical futility argue that physicians have a right to say, "Enough is enough!"

In an ominous move, Schneiderman and Jecker connect medical futility to the ends or goals of medicine, which for them also encompass "limits and terminations."[2] For them, healing the sick "is accomplished through assisting and working with nature."[3] All this sounds innocuous enough, until someone takes it out of the context of obviously terminal patients and attempts to generalize it to all of medicine. Then "natural" and "limits" become very restrictive.

Even with patients at the end of their lives, this is dangerous terrain, not nearly as solid as one might think. It has been very difficult in medical ethics to get consensus about actions in cases that are medically futile, and it is important to understand why.

First, judgments about medical futility may frequently mask judgments about *rationing*, cutting costs at the bedside by denying medical services. How does the family of a terminal patient know the physician's real motive, especially if he works for an HMO?

One of the most distressing stories I've heard about bioethics was told to me recently by an oncologist in a state dominated by HMOs. This oncologist had attended a conference about medical ethics and end of life sponsored by a large HMO, which had paid for various medical ethicists to speak to the oncologists about why giving futile treatment for cancer was not required and possibly unethical. The oncologist told me, "My HMO thought that if the ethicists sold their message, it would save it money on expensive, end-of-life care."

Of even greater interest, his large HMO employs bioethicists as consultants, who are (he claims) sometimes called in to convince a family that further medical intervention is futile. "When he walks on the ward," he told me, "he should be wearing black."

A second reason why medical futility is treacherous terrain is that those arguing for the right of physicians to stop futile treatment have, unfortunately, overestimated how eager people are to die. Consider the results of the SUP-PORT study, funded by billionaire George Soros as part of his "Dying in America" project.[4]

In it, the hypothesis was that if terminal patients better understood the futility of many interventions at the end of life, they would forsake such interventions and die more peacefully. Needless CPR, surgery, and misery could be avoided. Money could be saved. Specially trained clinical nurses intervened with patients who were given six months to live; they also intervened extensively with their families.

The nurses failed. They did not decrease the amount of CPR or futile medical treatment. While the physicians and oncology nurses had seen many similar patients with the same conditions for decades, the particular terminal disease was new to each patient coming in, and none wanted to just give up and die. As one angry woman replied, when asked by a SUPPORT nurse on admission about CPR and advanced directives, "I didn't come here to plan my death! I came here to beat cancer."[5] The SUPPORT study's failure to decrease futile interventions at the end of life suggests that, like organ donation, getting higher rates of success is not just a matter of educating people. There are deeper forces at work here.

Another reason for the failure is that patients and their families accepted degrees of misery that physicians and nurses thought intolerable. The medical staff didn't understand why patients and families didn't accept "death as a fact of life" and try to die with dignity. Of course, that's easy to say if you've seen the same disease a hundred times before and, more important, if you're not the one dying or the grieving spouse.

Similarly, another part of the SUPPORT study found that people who had previously signed advanced directives, stating they would rather die than live with a tracheotomy while being kept alive by a respirator, changed their minds when staring death in the face.[6] The average prediction in an advanced directive by competent patients about his own future wishes turned out to be inaccurate. Given a choice between a futile intervention but continued life and simply accepting that nothing else could be done and allowing death to occur, most choose the futile intervention.

Finally, it is widely known in internal medicine that many members of disadvantaged groups in U.S. society believe that "rationing" masquerades under the label of "futility." Ethnic patients, Medicaid patients, HMO patients with messy, chronic diseases, gay patients with HIV infections, and the families of these patients, do not always trust the medical system to do everything possible for the patient. And, in truth, physicians (who still tend to be white, heterosexual males) *do* like some patients more than others, and some of them *do* confuse rationing with futility.

Consider a case, variations on which I have heard several times around the country.[7] A white medical staff has told a black family that their eighty-four-year-old grandmother is dying, that further treatment is futile, and that they should let her die in peace. The grandmother has problems such as coronary artery disease, emphysema, or diabetes. The staff has resuscitated her several times, breaking bones in the process. It seems inhumane to the staff to put this frail old woman through this terrible process.

But the family and "Grandma Beverly" see things differently. The family was told treatment was futile a year ago, and told so by a white medical staff, and then Grandma Beverly did not die. They suspect that the staff secretly thinks it's not worthwhile for society to spend so much money on such an old black woman.

Grandma Beverly is religious, but does not want to go early. "God will take me when He is ready," she says. Her two remaining joys are the simple ones of going to church on Sunday morning and Wednesday evening, and going to the big indoor shopping mall. For each activity, she must use a motorized cart and breathe oxygen from a rolling canister, but she says she is happy. Neither she nor her family will sign a "DNR" (do not resuscitate) order. In this awkward state, Grandma Beverly lives two years after the first description of her condition as "medically futile." She spends her last six months in a nursing home, fighting death up to the last minute, enduring things that the staff say they would never undergo themselves.

This is the kind of case that haunts internal and geriatric medicine. It is frustrating, messy, and seemingly interminable. Israeli internist Shimon Glick has warned us that such treatments may be terminated early, ostensibly for the good of the patient, but really for the good of the medical staff, who want the case to end because the staff is confused, frustrated, and angry about its mistakes, disagreements, and inability to provide either a cure or a good death.[8]

In her comprehensive new book on medical futility, *When Doctors Say No*, bioethicist Susan Rubin mounts a devastating critique on the pervasive use of futility in modern medicine to cease treatment.[9] She argues that physicians are not trained to make judgments about evaluative futility ("it's not worth it") and don't share (as they should) such judgments with patients. Moreover, so-called factual futility or physiological futility is much more ambiguous, more evaluative than is commonly believed.

Rubin describes several telling examples—of a chronic alcoholic woman, of a child in persistent vegetative state whose parents want to care for him at home despite little chance of his ever waking up, and of an Oriental woman dying of liver cancer who wants to die for theological reasons in the right phase of the moon—where physicians and patients disagree about whether further treatment is futile.

More important, Rubin argues that where treatment is going to be denied because of medical futility, then such a reference to futility should not *stop* the discussion but *start* it. And the discussion should highlight the proposed, proper goals of medicine, bringing these out into the open for all to criticize, evaluate, accept, or reject.

Ironically, both Rubin, on one side, and Schneiderman and Jecker, on the other, agree that progress cannot occur without social discussion of, and subsequent agreement about, the proper goals of medicine. (This is also a conclusion pushed by bioethicist Daniel Callahan, which will be considered next.)

Because of this kind of case, and for the above-mentioned reasons, there is little likelihood that Americans will soon come to a consensus that physicians treating terminal patients should not provide futile treatment. If that is so for end-of-life treatment, how much more true will it be when people try to generalize futility beyond this narrow range? I now turn to this problem.

INTERLUDE: THE RIGHT AND THE GOOD

A very important distinction exists in ethics between personal life and public life. John Stuart Mill in his classic *On Liberty* called this the distinction between self-regarding and other-regarding actions. I shall follow many writers in using different terms for Mill's distinction and distinguish between a view of the good (or good life) and a view of morality. The former is personal and can be very private; the latter is necessarily public for it concerns actions that may harm others.

Although the distinction has rough edges, its broad concept is easy to understand. If a couple pays cash and contracts with a physician to help them overcome fertility, that is a decision that falls in personal life and within their theory of the good. Others may criticize them for wanting a baby so much, but there is no moral criticism that is justified because no one else is affected by their actions.

Suppose the man and the woman in the same couple both have HIV infections and desire to use modern techniques such as sperm washing and taking AZT to reduce the chances that any resulting baby will also be HIV infected. Now we have a moral issue, because a baby might be brought into the world with an infection that need not have occurred. It is also a moral issue because the costs of caring for such an HIV-infected baby over a lifetime, either by private or public medical coverage, could be quite high.

We can make such distinctions. A decision to buy a cellular phone is a personal, self-regarding decision; talking loudly on it in movie theaters, in waiting rooms of airports, and in the line at grocery stores is an immoral action because it harms others by disturbing their tranquility of thought and mood.

What makes modern civilization work, especially in democracies, is that we do not seriously try to dictate decisions about the good to others. I might think other people are making a mistake to be atheists, sports fanatics, or vegetarians, but so long as they leave me alone, I should leave them alone. If someone or some group tries to make me an atheist, or to compel me to watch sports continuously, or to forsake eating meat, then the personal-public distinction has been breached and their behavior is criticizable.

This distinction between the good and the right, as important as it is to allowing us all to actually get along, is constantly under attack by those on both the political Left and the Right. There are people who are very passionate about their view of the good and equate it with morality. They are omnimoralists and believe that anyone who fails to accept their theory of the good is harmed, for example, people who believe that if you do not accept their version of Christianity, you will go to Hell. Similarly, there are people who think that anyone who rejects their view of the family, sexual relations, or work is immoral and harms others by this rejection.

This is an old battle, one mostly won in real life, but still going on in education and politics where some want only "politically correct" values taught in school while others want only conservative "family values" taught. As any educated person knows, there are dozens of real theories of the good that people live by, and education cannot and should not endorse any of them (because we might be mistaken about which one is true, as Mill taught us).

This is basically the classic liberal view, although this label is confusing because Libertarians also endorse it and *liberal* means too many things to too many people today. I believe this view is the correct one for the same reason that Bertrand Russell defended democracy: it is not that so many great arguments can be given for it as that we know great arguments about why all the alternatives in history have led to disaster.

BROADENING FUTILITY: ACCEPTING NATURAL LIMITS

Astonishingly, there is a movement in bioethics to take natural limits far beyond medical futility and apply them to all of medicine. In this movement, medical futility at the end of life symbolizes such misguided attempts to go beyond natural limits. In the early 1970s Ivan Illich's influential *Medical Nemesis* argued that our medical system was actually "toxic" to our health, that individuals and their environments were chiefly responsible for health and disease, and that many of the problems of medicine stemmed from trying to exceed natural limits. Medicine then becomes dangerous, inhumane, exorbitant, and unnatural.[10]

In the 1980s, James Fries and Lawrence Crapo, two professors at Stanford Medical School, argued that "the median natural human life span is set at a maximum of 85 years with a standard error of less than one year. . . . In other words, one in 10,000 individuals reaches the age of 100."[11] The implications were obvious to them: "Immortality or superlongevity will not accrue to us."[12]

Between the lines, such authors suggest other messages: that high-tech medicine is attempting to transgress natural limits, that monies spent on the last years of life would better be spent on educating the young or on promoting social equality, and that medicine's goals need to be redirected toward accepting the inevitability of death and disease. At the beginning of the 1990s, Lee Goldman and Milton C. Weinstein at Harvard's School of Public Health offered a similar conclusion, namely, that human longevity is difficult to increase.[13]

A much more ambitious change is championed by Daniel Callahan. Callahan is one of the most famous bioethicists in the United States and one of the great pioneers of the field. More than thirty years ago in Hastings-on-Hudson, New York, he cofounded the Hastings Institute, the first interdisciplinary research think tank in medical ethics, and its bioethics journal, the *Hastings Center Report*. His early research and writing focused on abortion, reproductive issues, and death and dying. In the past decade, he has written a series of books that argue that there are definite limits to what medicine can do, that Americans should not be asked to pay endlessly for medical research, and that medicine should respect the natural rhythms and limits of life, not constantly try to change them.

In particular, Callahan thinks U.S. medicine extends human life past its natural boundaries with expensive technology: "We will not indefinitely continue to have the ability to pay for an expanding health care system, or for those endlessly emerging marvels of technology that promise to extend life."[14] In *What Kind of Life? The Limits of Medical Progress*, he writes that, "The very nature of medical progress is to pull to itself many more resources than can be of genuine benefit to many individuals, and much, much more than can be socially justifiable for the common good."[15] This is a remarkable indictment, one claiming that the very nature of medical progress has a kind of insidious harm in it. Instead of this false, future-looking conception of medical progress, Callahan likes a medicine that looks backward to simpler times:

> I have before my mind's eye a future healthcare system that seeks not to constantly conquer all disease and extend all life, but which seeks instead to enhance the quality of life; which seeks not always to overcome the failings and decline of the body, but helps people better accept and cope with them; which tries to keep in view that

health is a means to a decent life, not a value in its own right; which works to help
society curb its appetite for ever higher quality and constant improvements in
health care. It is a system that aims to intensify inward, seeking not the endless
conquests of all frontiers, but only those that promise a more coherent individual
life within a more coherent societal life.[16]

Callahan frequently laments the costs of medical treatment at the end of life,
the costs of assisted reproductive services purchased in cash by couples, and the
costs of continued medical research. In this he is like former Colorado Governor Richard Lamm, who writes,

Medical technology does not save us money, as a genre. "Cured" is a marvelous
word, but it also means "alive to die later of something else." We have reduced
mortality but dramatically increased morbidity. Where we used to die inexpen-
sively of the first or second disease, we now die expensively of the fifth or sixth disease, having consumed far more resources. A new world has formed. . . .
     We are thus left, in this strange and new world, with the task of deciding not
what is "beneficial" to a patient (which is a medical decision), but what is "appropriate" or "cost effective" (which is partly a social, economic, and a fairness decision). We have to balance quality of life with quantity of life, costs and benefits,
preventive medicine versus curative medicine. We are, unfortunately but realistically, into prioritizing medicine. Medicine will never be the same.[17]

It is important to note the running theme about society saving money in both
Lamm's and Callahan's remarks, as well as in many discussions of medical futility.
     I think that Lamm's and Callahan's vision is ultimately a dark and bleak one,
one telling us to cut back on medical research, that we are spending too much
on medicine. Importantly, Callahan and Lamm never specify exactly what percentage of the GNP is "too much" or what the opportunity cost is of slowing
down medical research.
     Some of us want a different medical system, one with the goals of eradicat-
ing all disease, reversing the decline of the body, extolling health as an intrinsic
value, and fulfilling the desires of society for medical progress, rather than
counseling people why they should not expect it.
     Before we give up too easily, note that researchers who say we can't increase
longevity are only talking about the results of eliminating chronic diseases, such
as heart disease and cancer, not about whether it is *biologically impossible* to increase longevity. Changes at the cellular level, where aging almost certainly begins, would offer new hope.
     One person who disagrees with this gloomy view is former chair of medicine
at Tufts University Medical School and current professor of medicine at the
University of Southern California, William B. Schwartz. He thinks that if med-

ical research concentrates in certain areas, then "conceivably by 2050, aging may in fact prove to be simply another disease to be treated."[18] It is commonly thought that normal cells can only divide about fifty times before rapid aging begins at the cellular level. This action is thought to be mediated by the telomeres at the caps of each chromosome. Each time cells divide, these telomeres get shorter and shorter, until the cap vanishes, and cellular death begins. (This is why the cloned lamb, Dolly, is thought to be older than she seems, because her telomeres may be shortened.) Schwartz and others think that research on telomerase, an enzyme natural to the body that has the ability to rebuild the caps on telomeres, could find a way to prevent such cellular death. Other research on the elimination of free radicals by natural antioxidants could achieve similar or better results. Already, researchers have discovered four genes that, when induced to mutate, allow roundworms to live almost five times longer than they normally would.[19]

Callahan wants to change our "understanding of a whole way of life" so that we can limit medicine and its costs. That is exactly why his view is dangerous: he wants to freeze us here in time, with no further progress, and to accept things as they are now. He would fund an egalitarian minimum of medical care for all through the lens of a communitarian ethos by denying expensive treatments to individuals at the end of life: no dialysis for Aunt Jane at eighty so the twenty-seven-year-old waiter can get medical coverage.[20]

It is a great mistake to think that a particular theory of the good (a.k.a. "the goals or ends of medicine") can solve the problems of morality. In his latest (1998) broadside, *False Hope: Why America's Quest for Perfect Health Is a Recipe for Failure*, Callahan himself offers just such a false hope:

> A medicine which says, in effect, that death and disease have no meaning and must simply be eliminated—in a society that says it can make no sense of them either and must abandon them to our hidden, private lives—is a medicine that offers no common rationale for sustainability. Everything is left to political process on the one hand, divorced from moral substance and depth, and to individual choice and direction on the other, sundered from any connection with a recognizable common good.[21]

Yet how can medicine itself say that death and disease have any meaning? Personally, I don't see any meaning to esophageal cancer or death. From a medical point of view, cancer is just uncontrolled cellular growth, molecular changes without meaning. Death and disease just happen, for no apparent reason. Would that they didn't.

Various religions try to give meaning to such terrible evils, which is to say, they claim that terminal disease does not afflict innocent people for no reason.

Instead, there are benevolent reasons why each seemingly evil thing happens to a particular person. But let's not confuse theistic solutions to the problem of evil with medical ethics for all of us.

Callahan writes, "A medicine that cannot anchor itself in any consensus about the nature of human needs, or the ends of human life, cannot set any coherent goals for itself."[22] When he so writes, he does a disservice to himself and to his readers, for he lets them think they have obtained an important insight, when in fact they have been befuddled by fancy words.

Yet medicine functions well today without agreement on a specific theory of the good. How? By the time-honored strategy of switching from content to process: medicine should have the "process goal" of giving patients first what they need and then what they want.

Callahan would limit medical progress by "a full scale examination of what constitutes the human good."[23] But the examination would be left largely skeletal (as in the works of Kass and Rifkin), because the more flesh it gets—the more cases appear of HIV patients, impaired babies, and those waiting for liver transplants—the more everyone sees how dramatically the determined human good differs from their own good. Not everyone embraces a quasi-religious quasi-fatalism conjoined with skepticism about paid reproductive assistance, physician-assisted dying, and the benefits of medical research.

Callahan thinks it terrible that we can't agree on the meaning of death and disease, because then "everything is left to political process." In this statement we hear the echo of the U.S. scholar Leo Strauss, a famous political elitist who constantly harped that modern political thinkers (and he would probably have said the same about today's bioethicists) cannot make important value judgments about the goals of society. Strauss endorsed the perfectionistic values of Plato and the ancient Greeks, which of course abhorred democracy and the ordinary person.

Despite Callahan and Strauss, political process is how democracy and real life work. What else is to be expected in a society where we have so many theories of how to live? Should we ban health food stores that sell herbs and products from complementary medicine? I don't agree with the values endorsed by the Golden Temple, but I don't want to ban its existence.

Over the past centuries, we have painfully evolved complex processes to live together peacefully with such divergent views. These processes are called "democracy," "the rule of law," and "morality."

A telling example is what Callahan wrote in 1990: "Whether it is intensive care for the premature newborn, low birth weight baby, bypass surgery for the very old, or AZT therapy for AIDS patients, the eventual outcome will not likely be good; and when those problems are solved, there will be others to take their place.[24] For Callahan, medicine should not focus on its "curative" function but on its "caring" function (a la hospice, when natural limits are accepted). Thankfully, medical research didn't heed this view and didn't accept HIV disease as a "natural limit" for HIV-infected people. Protease inhibitors have now transformed HIV infection to a quasi-stable condition, one no longer inexorably terminal.

Many people who write in bioethics and public policy assume that early, quick referral to hospice will save society money by forgoing expensive, high-tech, medical treatment. They would substitute an "ethics of care"—which they presume is cheap—for an "ethics of treatment"—which they presume is futile. But evidence suggests that good hospice care, with attention to real relief of pain and adequate psychiatric support, is not cheap at all and will save no money whatsoever.[25] If hospice is to be preferred, it should be preferred for reasons other than saving money.

Ultimately for Callahan, medicine can do little in the face of disease and death:

> Now, if we agree that there is evil in the pain and suffering brought on by biological causes, what kind of evil is it? Even if some of the evil is avoidable, much of it is not and never will be. It is simply part of the way things are. In that case, medicine would do well to understand that its task must be to help people live with that evil, not fool themselves into thinking that it can someday be utterly eliminated.[26]

Translation: God wants you to suffer; accept it.

WHAT IS HEALTH?

In 1947, the World Health Organization (WHO) redefined health in a remarkable way, "Health is a state of complete physical, mental, and social well-being and not merely the absence of disease or infirmity." What a wonderful definition of health for medicine! This definition implies that health is not just a negative, as the absence of something, but a positive, evolving state.

But a positive state can be defined as the average functioning of a people at a certain time and place in history or as an ideal to be approached, which itself improves over centuries.

Many critics think the WHO definition is incorrect because one can be happy without being healthy and because being healthy doesn't guarantee being happy.[27] Well, of course! But also talk to the millions of formerly unhappy people now on Prozac and Zoloft. Suppose these two happiness drugs are just the tip of the iceberg. What's the retort? Force people to accept natural limits and be naturally miserable? Stop hip replacements?

Such critics think that human desire is elastic and infinite, such that the more medicine gives us, the more we will want. True, but so what? A hundred years ago, if people were given the means to live to be seventy-five instead of thirty-five, they would have jumped at the chance. Like us, they would want to live to be a hundred. People want lots of life, fun, love, and exciting experiences. Most people for most of history have not, and perhaps never will, get enough of these. More is better; limits are bad.

ENHANCEMENT AND IMPROVEMENT

Urging anyone to accept natural limits is a dangerous precedent in medicine. Giving up, saying it's "futile" to continue, and urging patients to sign DNR orders to save society money should be limited to carefully chosen cases, not generalized to the goals of medicine.

Take an example from sports. As seen, Schneiderman and Jecker agree with Callahan. They argue that medicine must agree about the proper ends it serves in order to function properly and to agree about what is improper functioning (and hence, often futile). They argue that enhancing athletic powers is not a proper medical goal or benefit:

> In our view, the [for a physician to give an athlete an] anabolic steroid is futile because it does not provide any medical benefit to patients in the first place. After all, *enhancing athletic prowess is not a medical goal*; rather, medicine is concerned with restoring health and healing the patient. Giving an athlete large doses of steroids certainly does not make a sick person well, nor does it rehabilitate a handicapped person to a level of ordinary functioning. There was a notorious time in recent history when Nazi doctors aspired to make a super-race by selectively breeding those they thought possessed superior qualities and exterminating those they thought lacked such qualities. But this goal, which violates the fundamental duty of beneficence to every patient, never has been part of the historical tradition of medicine. Nor does the ethical practice of medicine embrace such a goal today.[28] (my emphasis)

This quotation is actually amazing and illuminating. Notice that as soon as we depart from the "proper" goals of medicine, we are Nazis. In this expansive definition of futility, pursuing any divergent theory of the good becomes medically futile.

This is quite a dramatic claim. Vast, new areas of medicine are now relegated to the label "improper." Plastic surgery that aims to improve appearance, rather than restoring it after disfigurement, is improper. Sports medicine that aims to improve performance, rather than to treat injuries, is improper. Psychiatric consultation that aims to extract the most from life, rather than merely to treat mental illness, is improper. Of course, it almost goes without mention for the above critics that genetic enhancements are improper goals for medicine.

The same kind of somatic genetic therapy that could give a crippled adult a missing protein so he could walk might also be used to help a good athlete become a great one. Once genetic tools work that change dysfunction into normal functioning, those same tools will in different contexts be usable to elevate normal functioning to great functioning.

Take sports, which some critics say will be destroyed by drugs and genetic enhancements.[29] Is this criticism on target? I don't think so. For me the point of sports is not to take primitive humans as they are at some fixed point in time and then see how well they can compete. Sports have no one point, and different goals may emerge for different people. Just as there are different kinds of competitions for adult men and women, for kids by age group, and for professionals and amateurs, there is no intrinsic reason why there cannot be competitive sports for enhanced athletes.

One goal of any physical activity is not to beat everybody else, but to see how far you can push yourself. If a person can only compete in the Iditarod on drugs, or with genetic enhancements, then let us have a special Super Iditarod for such athletes (already the dogs, the *real* athletes in the race, have been bred for generations from special lines of racing dogs).

All the arguments in medicine about "natural limits," "frivolous services," and "wasteful treatments" will soon be applied to bodily and mental enhancements. One can see the debate coming. Just as some will say that physicians have no business doing facelifts, so they will say that physicians should not increase the strength of athletes or the memory of scholars. Some now say that psychiatrists should not waste their time helping rich clients understand themselves when insane inmates of mental institutions have no psychiatrist at all.

Nothing that has been said so far applies to what forms of medical services should be subsidized by government or large group coverage plans. Such forms of subsidy may not choose to cover enhancements, just as they may not cover cosmetic plastic surgery today or psychotherapy for personal growth. The specific philosophical question in contention here is whether a new kind of medicine, one that goes far beyond curing disease and rehabilitating patients and aggressively tries to help people become better, is proper and good. Is this "Nazi medicine" or a proper part of a new medicine?

ONUS OF PROOF

Before going further, let's talk about onus-of-proof arguments. Generally, you want the onus of proof on the other side. This is one of those "first steps" discussed throughout this book, that is, how the parameters of a debate in medical ethics get conceptualized.

So far, the onus of proof has been on those who would seek to exceed "natural" limits. Because medicine has had few tools with which to work, such seeking has been to date largely theoretical. But as we enter the twenty-first century, and a new world of genetic possibilities, we need to rethink this issue and how it is set up.

So let's reverse the onus of proof by asking: *Why should there be any limits at all on what a competent adult can ask a physician to do to her body?* Should there be any limits at all on what risks a competent man can take with somatic genetic enhancements? At present we allow people to try to scale Mt. Everest, even though the highest trails are littered with the frozen dead bodies of previous climbers who have failed. At present, we allow people to invest all their savings in a start-up business where they hope to make millions, even though most small businesses fail.

If we were talking about making changes in the germ line, about changes in genes that could be passed down over generations, then moral questions could arise because future children would be affected. But so long as competent adults only change their somatic cells, which cannot be passed on to the next generation (at least, without cloning, which is another question), then no other person will be directly affected.

If we were talking about making changes and billing the public or group plans for medical coverage, then questions would arise of public policy, of just allocation of scarce resources. But if such changes are paid for in cash by competent adults, with an adult negotiating the services of a physician-scientist, then no questions arise involving public monies.

I think the onus of proof should be on those who would impose any kind of limits on adults wanting to enhance themselves. How the onus of proof gets set up is important, because if it is on those wanting to enhance themselves, it will be very difficult for them to justify the need for any change.

Limitations on optional medical services are like limitations on free speech and ideas. As John Stuart Mill taught us in *On Liberty*, when the government, the majority, and conservative medical opinion decide that certain kinds of goods are allowed but not others, there is a good chance that they will decide incorrectly. For example, in 1976, the American Medical Association (AMA) considered removing a respirator from a comatose Karen Quinlan to be "euthanasia"; five years later, it said removing respirators was permissible but condemned removing feeding tubes from such patients; today the AMA accepts removing life-sustaining treatment but condemns physician-assisted dying for terminal patients.[30] In all these instances, the evaluative judgments of most physicians were incorrect and behind the times.

Should something go wrong, for example, a mathematician gets a brain tumor from taking massive doses of a cognition-enhancing drug, then he will be like the stunt driver who takes the money to jump his motorcycle over a canyon: he pays with his own body and life. That is easy to understand. What is not easy to understand is how a physician can be such an expert on theories of the good life that he knows which lifestyles are to be allowed and which are not. Certainly there is no training in medical school or medicine that imparts such wisdom.

PHYSICIANS AS GATEKEEPERS OF THE GOOD LIFE?

When it comes to deciding what is allowed for patients or what improvements are frivolous, physicians are indisputably our society's gatekeepers. They alone are licensed to provide medical services and prescribe drugs. The U.S. system operates on that assumption. So much so that here it is easier to get a handgun than a prescription.

As gatekeepers, physicians are told to be Solomon-like in denying "unnecessary" services desired by patients. Everyone would agree that physicians should deny patients who would harm other people, for example, a fleeing criminal who wants plastic surgery to escape capture, a young male who wants the "date rape" drug (gamma hydroxbutyrate, a.k.a. "GHB") to use to sexually assault unconscious young women. But how far should such denials go when patients desire services that will not harm others but only themselves? What if the harm to themselves is not certain, but likely? What if it is only possible?

Harm is not a factual word, although it is frequently taken to be so in medical contexts. *Harm* covers a continuum, from the mere offense of someone forgetting your name to the deadly injury of torture. A yearlong course in law school—torts—covers the array of harms that humans inflict on one another, as well as means of redress.

Consider the controversy about use of anabolic steroids (androstenedione) in competitive sports such as weight lifting and bodybuilding. Here the person using the drugs is not a patient but a client who wishes to improve his body. Because the physician is the gatekeeper, he must make the key evaluative judgments.

But these evaluative judgments differ dramatically from those of morality. Here the physician doesn't try to prevent harm of one person to another but either tries to prevent harm to a client based on the physician's particular theory of the good or rejects altogether the patient's differing theory of the good.

Some people consider use of anabolic steroids harmful and would ban their use in all sports. (Because the use of water-based steroids in training can be stopped before big events, and are then undetectable in urine tests, such bans may be difficult to enforce. Also, there are thousands of variations of such steroids, and each test detects only a specific molecular form.) Certainly athletes need information informing them of proven harms from long-term use.

Some opposition to giving steroids is not based on a concern for the long-term health of athletes but on a quite different evaluative judgment that competitive sports should be natural, that athletes should not use drugs to improve performance, and that athletes should not be biologically enhanced to compete. These are highly evaluative judgments.

In making them, ordinary citizens and physician-gatekeepers condemn not just theoretical views of the good life *but views actually lived by people*. If a person closely identifies with such an ideal, condemning his ideal is very close to condemning him. To say that bulking up your body should not be so important to you, that you should also acquire an interest in poetry or computers, is patronizing. It is to imply that you are childish, immature, and need a physician to be your "pater."

Suppose use of such drugs carries some but not a great risk (as it may be in low-to-moderate dosages, carefully monitored). Does it follow that physicians should refuse such drugs on the grounds that their use falls within the category "improper" goals of humans? Suppose, for example, that the worst possibility of using steroids is a 10 percent chance of getting liver cancer. Now liver cancer is a very bad result and not easily curable, and most people would not want to run such a risk.

But suppose some do. What is the proper goal of medicine here? Surely, a minimal goal is to make sure the patient (or "client") achieves real informed consent about the dangers of using such drugs. After that, is it a proper goal of medicine to judge that this risk is (as in some judgments of medical futility) "not worth it"? Is paternalism about another's life plans justified here? About another's theory of the good?

One way of looking at this question is whether (in the assumed, worst-case scenario, which might be much too dire) it is reasonable for physicians to allow patients to take a 10 percent risk of death from services the physicians could choose to withhold. For those who think that it is reasonable to do so, consider another common situation in medicine where the opposite kind of risk gets the common endorsement of physicians.

In cases of esophageal, liver, or lung cancer in adults over sixty, the chances of living five years after diagnosis by the combined use of surgery, chemotherapy, and radiation could be as low as 10 percent. Moreover, if the patient opts for this combined treatment, the chances are also very high that he will die a worse death than he would if he were to opt for palliative care. (He would suffer the terrible trauma of major surgery—which most people underestimate before they've gone through it—likely radiation burns, and the sickness, nausea, and lack of appetite caused by the chemotherapy. On top of all this, he would experience an enormous tiredness and lack of energy.) Despite such terrible odds, it is thought reasonable to let a patient risk a 90 percent chance of a worse death to try for a 10 percent or less chance of (at best) a five-year cure. It seems that a particular theory of the good is most favored in medicine, one that hangs on to every thread of life through enormous suffering and effort.

The point here is not to judge one person's theory of the good (risk taking) over another's, but to emphasize the asymmetry in viewing what patients request of physicians. When patients follow the traditional path, questionable choices are allowed and even encouraged. When patients go along a new path, it seems they must justify themselves every inch of the way.

Although many people will not be sympathetic with this example, if we let the desire to bulk up one's muscles stand for similar "biological" (as opposed to "behavioral") enhancements, we will see that wider issues are at stake. The coming years will likely bring many possible genetic enhancements that competent adults will be willing to risk some danger to themselves in order to get. Medicine is not adverse to risk taking (consider the risks of bypass surgery), so the question will arise, "What gives physicians the moral authority to decide that certain kinds of risk taking are 'wrong' or not part of the 'proper' role of medicine?" There are certainly no "ethical OSCEs" (moral tests) in medical school, such that only certifiably ethical medical students become physicians. Nor do medical students get any training in medical school about which theories of the good are reasonable and defensible and which are not.

Most likely, U.S. medicine will be conservative and stick its head in the sand, forcing those who want such enhancements to go abroad or underground. But is that a good thing? Maybe some real, valuable genetic enhancements will come along that we should subject to randomized clinical trials or at least, study on a case-by-case basis.

ENDS OF MEDICINE AND THEORIES OF THE GOOD

One interesting question concerns whether belief in God should figure into the proper ends of medicine. Many people think that if God exists, then it affects how humans should conduct themselves, and from that it would seem to follow also that, if God exists, his existence affects how medicine should be conducted and how physicians should treat patients. For example, a deeply religious Christian, Jewish, or Hindu physician is urged not to see medicine as a way of amassing wealth but as a way of life dedicated to serving the sick.

So the philosophical question of whether God exists directly confronts one of the most essential questions about "the" goals of medicine: What is the goal of the good physician? A life of service or a life of personal achievement?

Consider related questions of whether patients have souls, whether there is an afterlife, and whether there is a spiritual dimension of healing achieved through supernatural intervention in the form of prayer, miracles, and talismans. If all these exist, then spiritual healers should have a proper place inside hospitals and should be incorporated into the medical team from the very beginning.

Is it a proper goal of medicine to decide which religious beliefs matter and which do not? That religions like Jehovah's Witnesses, Christian Scientists, and Scientologists are "cults," but Freewill Baptists, Seventh-Day Adventists, Mormons, and ultraorthodox Jews are not? Yet what more could define a person's view of the good life, his theory of the good, than acceptance of such a creed?

These religious questions are only the beginning of many conflicts within medicine about its proper goals. Politically, one must ask whether medicine should be elitist or egalitarian. Should our goal be to make America's physicians like China's barefoot doctors, where the physician is on the same social status as his clients, or should we continue the present system, with the great social gap between physicians and patients? What about distribution of medical benefits? Is proper medicine committed to a national, single-payer system run by the government? Or is the proper goal of medicine a Libertarian one?

Is it a proper goal of medicine to be committed to politically correct views? What if evidence accumulates that certain behaviors between men and women are really hardwired into the brain and genes, not amenable to change by social environment? Is it a proper goal of medicine to accept or reject biological sexism? What about racial or ethnic differences?

These questions are certainly social, moral, political, and important for public policy and the law, but how much are they amenable to defense as "the" proper goals of medicine? I think very little. And the more specific we get about particular visions of the good life, the less medicine has any moral authority to make judgments: Is being single a valuable life or an inferior one? Is it necessary to have a family to have the best life? A good job? A career that spans one's whole life and builds upon itself, stage-by-stage? How important is a robust sex life in the good life? Is it a proper or improper goal of medicine to help people achieve such a sex life? For gay men and lesbians too? What about them as parents?

In my own view, medicine is ultimately just a kind of knowledge that society allows some of its members to obtain. Knowledge in itself is neutral as to the goals it serves. Knowledge is a tool that can be used for good or bad, moral or evil, purposes. As such, it is what the Oxford philosopher Gilbert Ryle called a "category mistake" to think that there are certain evaluative goals that are part of knowledge itself. To believe so is like believing a knife can only be used to cut food at a table and never to harm humans, or to believe that an intravenous line can be used in a hospital only to help patients and never to harm them.

It follows that we will never make progress by trying to figure out the proper goals of "knife using" or "IV-drip using." The proper goals of these tools are not dictated by the tools themselves but by the things human want in using them. Deciding "the" proper goals of medicine, whether about futility, medical research, or enhancement, amounts to deciding what humans need and want, which puts us back at where we started.

CONCLUSIONS

So long as the client is a competent adult paying cash for anticipated medical services, why should any limits be put on what is "proper medicine"? Given that marathon running is a joy to one person and an agony to another, why should anyone judge which is better?

One is reminded of the silly debate in the 1980s about whether competent HIV-infected patients should be allowed to try risky, experimental therapies for AIDS. Given no other alternatives and likely death, the debate seems silly now, yet few such patients were allowed to do so.[31]

To invoke "natural" to stop medical progress is dangerous. *Natural* can be just another name in medicine for *fatalistic* and *primitive*. To say that we should not spend so much on medical research, because medicine is consuming more and more of our GNP, is not in itself an argument against such expenditures. Who is to say that 10, 20, or 30 percent of the GNP or personal income is "too much" to spend on medical care? Let the political process decide not a priori speculation.

Medical advancement can reshape what it means to be human: better athletes through enhancement medicine, brighter and funnier children through cloning, and three careers instead of one-plus-retirement as longevity increases. Medical discoveries such as broad-spectrum antibiotics in the mid-1940s eradicated a whole class of bacterial diseases. Our contemporary naysayers imply that the years of such discoveries are in the past.

I am more optimistic. Exploding knowledge about molecular genetics is giving us new opportunities, if not for ourselves, then for the next generation. Talk of futility—at the bedside, for the goals of medicine, or vis-à-vis medical research—is often premature.

NOTES

1. Lawrence J. Schneiderman and Nancy Jecker, *Wrong Medicine: Doctors, Patients, and Futile Treatment* (Baltimore, Md.: Johns Hopkins University Press, 1995).

2. Ibid., 5.

3. Ibid., 130.

4. SUPPORT Principal Investigators, "A Controlled Trial to Improve Care for Seriously Ill Hospitalized Patients: The Study to Understand Prognoses and Preferences for Outcomes and Risks of Treatments (SUPPORT)," *Journal of the American Medical Association* 274, nos. 20, 22 (29 November 1995): 1591–8.

5. Renee Oliverio and Beth Fraulo, "SUPPORT Revisited: The Nurse Clinician's Perspective," *Holistic Nursing Practice* (October 1998): 1.

6. Teno J. et al. "Advance Directives for Seriously Ill Hospitalized Patients: Effectiveness with the Patient Self-Determination Act and the SUPPORT Intervention. SUPPORT Investigators. Study to Understand Prognoses and Preferences for Outcomes and Risks of Treatment," *Journal of American Geriatric Society* 45, no. 4 (April 1997): 500–507; Teno J. et al. "Do Advance Directives Provide Instructions that Direct Care? SUPPORT Investigators. Study to Understand Prognoses and Preferences for Outcomes and Risks of Treatment," *Journal of American Geriatric Society* 45, no. 4 (April 1997): 508–12.

7. I have heard this case and ones similar to it described many times. One such time was by bioethicist Henry Perkins at his Grand Rounds talk at UAB in 1997.

8. Shimon Glick, "Euthanasia: An Unbiased Decision?" *American Journal of Medicine* 102, no. 3 (March 1997): 294–6.

9. Susan Rubin, *When Doctors Say No: The Battleground of Medical Futility* (Bloomington: Indiana University Press, 1998).

10. Ivan Illich, *Medical Nemesis: The Expropriation of Health* (New York: Random House, 1976).

11. James Fries and Lawrence Crapo, *Vitality and Aging: Implications of the Rectangular Curve* (San Francisco: W. H. Freeman, 1981), 76–7.

12. Ibid., 139.

13. Knight Ridder News Service, "Heart Disease, Life Span Studied," *Birmingham Post-Herald*, 15 April 1991, A7. Reporting on an article by Lee Goldman and Milton C. Weinstein in the April 1991 issue of *Circulation*.

14. Daniel Callahan, *What Kind of Life? The Limits of Medical Progress* (New York: Simon and Shuster, 1990), 19.

15. Ibid., 21.

16. Ibid., 22–3.

17. Richard D. Lamm, "St. Martin of Tours in a New World of Medical Ethics," *Cambridge Quarterly of Healthcare Ethics* 3 (1994): 159–67. Reprinted in *Classic Works in Medical Ethics*, ed. Gregory Pence (New York: McGraw-Hill, 1995), 358, 364.

18. William B. Schwartz, *Life without Disease: The Pursuit of Medical Utopia* (Berkeley: University of California Press, 1998), 153.

19. E. Pennisi, "Premature Aging Gene Discovered," *Science* 272, no. 5259, (1996): 193–4; E. Pennisi, "Worm Genes Imply a Master Clock," *Science* 272, no. 5264 (1996): 949–50.

20. Daniel Callahan, *False Hope: Why America's Quest for Perfect Health Is a Recipe for Failure* (New York: Simon and Schuster, 1998), 28.

21. Ibid., 287.

22. Ibid.

23. Ibid.

24. Callahan, *What Kind of Life?*, 63.

25. Ezekiel Emanuel, "Cost Savings at the End of Life: What Do the Data Show?" *New England Journal of Medicine* 275, no. 24 (26 June 1996): 1907–14.

26. Callahan, False *Hope,* 286.

27. Callahan, *What Kind of Life?*, 39, 55.

28. Schneiderman and Jecker, *Wrong Medicine,* 5.

29. Sharon Begley, "The Real Scandal," *Newsweek* (15 February 1999): 48–54. I am indebted to a discussion on the MCW-listserv in late August 1996 about the subject of drugs, competitive sports, and enhancements.

30. Gregory E. Pence, "Comas," *Classic Cases in Medical Ethics: Accounts of the Cases that Shaped Medical Ethics,*" third edition (New York: McGraw-Hill, 2000), chapter 2.

31. See Udo Schuklenk's *Terminal Patients and Experimental Life-Saving Therapies* (London: Haworth, 1997).

RE-CREATING BIOETHICS

Our subject here is the performance of philosophers—"ethicists"—as commentators on public events. Sometimes they do what we might think philosophers ought to do: challenge the prevailing orthodoxy, calling into question the assumptions that people unthinkingly make. But just as often they function as orthodoxy's most sophisticated defenders, assuming that the existing social consensus must be right and articulating its theoretical "justification."

—James Rachels, "When Philosophers Shoot from the Hip," in *Can Ethics Provide Answers?*

In the twenty-seven years I have been involved with bioethics, it has grown from being a toddler who could barely crawl, to an awkward adolescent unsure of who he wants to be, and finally to a self-conscious adult.[1] The inception of the modern field of bioethics can be fixed in several ways. University of Washington bioethicist Albert Jonsen takes it to be 1967, with the publicity about Seattle's "God Committee" and its decisions about who should live and who should die based on who would get a hemodialysis machine. Others would count as the key event the origination of the Hastings Center and its *Report* in 1971.

As the twenty-first century begins, some of the founders of bioethics (such as Jonsen) are retiring, writing histories of bioethics, and preparing the way for new blood. During these decades, a few bioethicists have become very famous, making "medical ethicist" a familiar phrase to educated Americans. There are other signs of growth: the new American Association for Bioethics and the Humanities (ASBH) has a thousand members. Most medical schools require at least a few hours of medical ethics.[2] With college students, bioethics has been one of the fastest-growing courses of recent decades. In England, the General Medical Council has stressed the need for teaching medical ethics at both the undergraduate and postgraduate levels.[3]

Yet all is not completely well within the kingdom. Looking in from the outside, the average American might see signs of dissent, like ancient Greek peasants looking up at Mt. Olympus, unable to see the gods but seeing their presence in smoke, fire, and thunder. Bioethicists move from institution to institution; some are fired; some hunger for grants; others disdain applying. Where once only philosophers held forth, waves of M.D.-clinical ethicists are storming the foothills, fighting uphill for new positions and each year staking out new territory. But "Ph.D. only bioethicists" (as some M.D.-bioethicists refer to them) are not without their own new recruits, as hundreds of new Ph.D.s seek teaching jobs and write about bioethics (followed, in turn, by thousands of undergraduates who would like to do the same).

Whither will bioethics go? Right now, two kinds of bioethics have evolved, each competing for the title of the "real" bioethics. This chapter discusses the differences between these two kinds, mentions some conflicts between them, and then suggests a compromise. In this discussion, *bioethics* and *medical ethics* are used synonymously.

TWO KINDS OF BIOETHICISTS

Whatever the origins, bioethics has been around for at least thirty years and by now has developed some distinct styles. I will distinguish between "inside" and "outside" bioethicists, who sometimes think about bioethics in different ways.

As the name implies, inside bioethicists work inside medicine. They attempt to understand the facts of clinical cases and get the right answers to difficult clinical situations that raise ethical dilemmas. They often serve on hospital ethics committees (HECs) and may even be consulting bioethicists. Increasingly, inside bioethicists are "clinical" ethicists who hold M.D. degrees.

In contrast, outside bioethicists work parallel to medicine, or outside of it. They are not focused primarily on getting cases to turn out well. Instead, they are more interested in understanding the global questions facing medicine. They are more interested in where medicine is going, especially where it should go, than in helping particular physicians solve day-to-day cases. They discuss issues such as genetic discrimination, rights of animals in medical research, and the justice of systems of medical finance. Outside ethicists are "big picture" thinkers.

As Al Jonsen emphasizes, "Thirty years ago, all bioethicists were outsiders."[4] Then, an ethicist in medicine was one who wanted to discuss publicly what hitherto had only been discussed privately. University of North Carolina lawyer-bioethicist Nancy King agrees, "One of the original roles for people in bioethics was the 'outsider,' the moral stranger, the one who tried to help others find their voices."[5]

Outside bioethicists need not work outside the medical system, and indeed, some of the best work inside medical schools, but most outside ethicists work outside hospitals.[6] Most outside bioethicists are affiliated with universities or institutes.

Outside bioethicists are asked to give papers at other institutions on topics such as rights of animals, a right to medical care, abortion, or the concept of personhood in bioethics. Inside bioethicists are asked to give talks on topics such as medical futility, withdrawal of medical treatment from incompetent, dying patients, and informed consent.

There is a danger in only being an inside bioethicist. One can get too caught up with trying to understand and apply the norms inside medicine and too rarely step back and criticize those norms. Some well-known inside ethicists mimic the positions of most physicians on the controversial moral issues of our time, such as physician-assisted dying, gene therapy, surrogate mothers, the Ayala case (the girl conceived so that there would be a source for a bone marrow transplant for her older sister), human cloning, and assisted reproduction. Doing this too much raises the question of what the unique function of a medical ethicist is. After all, almost any physician can give the current opinions of most physicians on a particular moral issue, and this is also one job the AMA does well.

Understandably, working inside a hospital or medical school makes one attuned to the needs and crises there, not to the larger philosophical scene. Carl Elliot, who has both Ph.D. and M.D. degrees and who teaches at the University of Minnesota, writes:

> When bioethics is driven solely by clinical concerns, usually those of the hospital, it runs the danger of getting stuck in a permanent feedback loop in which the same issues are discussed again and again: informed consent, termination of life-sustaining treatment, patient confidentiality, brain death, surrogate decision-making, and most recently, the concept of medical futility. Constrained by the demand for immediately useful answers, clinical ethics (at its worst, at any rate) comes dangerously close to being a purely technical enterprise carried out in isolation from any deep reflection about the examined life, the way lives ought to be lived, and the way they ought to end.[7]

There is a widespread misconception that inside medical ethicists are moral experts and, because of their superior moral insights and training, they give "the" right answer to ordinary physicians befuddled by the deep ethical dilemmas they encounter. (Not only do ethicists not have such answers, but even if they did, few physicians would be willing to receive the answers from them). For example, in an October 1999 overview article in the *British Medical Journal* on medical ethics as a career, one physician-journalist characterized such U.S. medical ethicists as:

> The U.S. ethicists lurk around the hospital armed with a bleeper [sic] waiting to be called whenever a moral dilemma crops up. They may be given as little as 15 minutes to provide the definitive ethical answer on problems such as whether to remove the organs from a brain dead patient or if a 12 year old child has the right to refuse lifesaving surgery.[8]

(Admittedly, this article is written in the customary, patronizing tone of English/European writers of "Oh-look-what-those-silly-crass-warmongering-Americans-came-up-with-now"; nevertheless, it is amazing that the physician thinks her description accurately portrays hospital-based medical ethicists. [I know of no American bioethicist in a hospital who is actually called upon to give such answers in such an on-the-spot way.])

Danger also exists in only being an outside medical ethicist. If one writes about moral issues in medicine and never submits one's analysis to the test of real cases, or to the withering criticisms of physicians who deal with the same kind of cases each month, there is a sense in which one is only playing a theoretical game. To be real and truthful, ethics must meet real people in their conundrums and messy complexity. We can talk all day about how the system "ought" to be, for example, that the United States should have universal medical coverage like Canada, but physicians may still need to know if it is permissible to deceive insurance companies to get poor patients adequate care by "upcoding."[9]

It is the nature of the beast that inside medical ethicists seek consensus for their opinions. Ideally, they would like to speak with one voice, such that the same ethicist would say the same thing in identical clinical situations. This is the idea behind the recent push to develop "core competencies" among bioethics consultants. When inside ethicists get together, on panels or doing consultations, they strive to present the same face to the world.

Inside ethicists thus mimic physicians in cultivating a sense of professionalism. "That isn't a *professional* opinion in medical ethics," one inside ethicist says to another at a national meeting. The assumption was that one professional opinion did indeed exist about the subject (in this case, physician-assisted dying, which the ethicist opposed).

What is good about this approach is that such a consensus usually is achieved by carefully considering many different points of view. Indeed, the consensus of such bioethicists is usually not about content but about a process of achieving acceptable results. So they recommend ways to help physicians and families achieve good deaths through processes such as advanced directives, do-not-resuscitate orders, informed consent, ethics committees, and communication with patients as an ongoing affair, not as a one-time event. As such, it is rare for inside bioethicists to advocate an extreme point of view, especially one about content ("all patients in persistent vegetative state should be considered brain dead and organ donors") but they commonly advocate ways to achieve a fair process.

Inside ethicists are most likely found in the Society for Bioethics Consultation. Most, but not all, physician ethicists (also known as "clinical medical ethicists") are inside bioethicists. In this particular subset of inside ethicists, the goal is reimbursement for ethics consultation in hospitals.

Inside bioethicists frequently apply for and receive grants. This means they are subject to peer review, especially for grants from the federal government. Because inside bioethicists are almost exclusively reviewers of such grants, inside bioethicists are exquisitely sensitive to what other inside bioethicists think and write about.

One of the dangers of inside bioethics crops up here. Privately, almost all bioethicists doubt whether much has been accomplished by federal funding of bioethics, most famously in the Ethical, Legal, and Social Issues (ELSI) arm of the Human Genome Project (HGP). ELSI has been lavishly funded with 2 percent of the HGP money, and a lot of money has gone to some programs. But so far, there appear to have been far too many talks at public libraries, conferences, and surveys—few of which have moved the field along. A famous bioethicist remarked a year or so ago that no one could think of any really good paper or study that had been funded by ELSI.

It is not that there are not talented, smart people getting grants. It is rather that the process of getting grants is time-consuming and cumbersome, and considering the time it takes them to go through the whole process of applying, they could often have written the article the grant was meant to support.

Most practicing physicians, even in medical centers, see bioethics as an inside affair. They have little patience for thinking outside the box of their professional concerns. But this myopia condemns them to never getting outside of their own point of view. As the previous quotation from Carl Elliot mentions, most ethics rounds go nowhere. They remain discussions of the same issues with new cases, but never achieving any advances. After attending one or two of these sessions, it is easy for a physician to conclude, "Bah, bioethics! What's the point? They never get anywhere." True, enough, but who sets up this box, anyway?

Consider, too, the paradox that the definition of *malpractice* is often defined as departure from the reasonable and normal standards of physicians in one's community. Now there's a tight box for medical ethics, for how can progress ever occur without departure from antiquated standards? And does the first enlightened physician who so departs commit "malpractice"? (Such questions are never discussed.)

KNOWLEDGE AND TWO KINDS OF BIOETHICISTS

Professionalism and reimbursed consultation require the existence of a body of knowledge and a consensus on standards for interpreting it. Whether such a body of knowledge exists is a flash point between these two kinds of bioethicists.

Paradoxically, both inside and outside bioethicists may agree that such a body of knowledge exists but disagree dramatically over what it is. One is reminded here of Stephen Toulmin's famous essay, "The Tyranny of Principles," in which he noted that all the scholars on the president's commission agreed that certain things were wrong, say, psychosurgery on prisoners without their consent, but disagreed violently on the principles explaining *why* each thing was wrong.[10]

Outside bioethicists tend to think that theoretical issues are very important to doing bioethics well. Some of the most arcane outside bioethicists roam the airy halls of philosophy graduate departments, where theories of bioethics rarely touch a real case. This is "applied" ethics only in a metaphorical sense. Such outside bioethicists may spend many years writing about principles, intuitions, and made-up cases. Inspired by "pure philosophers" in ethical theory, such as Judith Jarvis Thomson, Derek Parfit, and Francis Kamm, they are not really as concerned with advancing medical practice as they are with producing elegant works of abstract ethical reflection.

By far the dominant kind of use of theory by outside bioethicists is the methodology of "applying" theories to a case to arrive at the correct answer. This methodology is often taught to beginners in bioethics, especially in undergraduate courses or one-shot lectures in medical school.

If there is anything that makes inside bioethicists bristle, it is the idea of "applying" ethical theories to real cases to get the right answers. Inside bioethicists minimally believe that applications of such theories and principles are intellectually bankrupt. They believe, often from hard experience with real cases or on ethics committees, that no theory, combination of theories, or set of principles can be "applied" to a case in order to crank out a right answer.

There is also a stronger claim. Applied to students, this is the claim that such a methodology actually makes them worse off. Like the Sophists of old, the theorists harm their students by teaching them to believe something false when previously the students believed something true. Students entered class thinking they could make good judgments in ethics or bioethics without knowing anything about ethical theories. After class, they leave thinking that this is false. Of course, they still don't understand how to use theory to get the right answers, but they assume that must be their own fault. If only they knew more theory, some assume, they could always get the right answer (like their professors, whose carefully chosen examples give the appearance that they always know the answers). In this the students are like people who get a taste of Gnosticism and wish they had been initiated to the secrets of the inner circle.

Some outside bioethicists use ethical theory the same way, as a kind of professional crutch to explain the distinctive contribution of philosophers to medical ethics ("Theories 'R Us"). We may not know much about medical facts or about how medicine works, but we know theories, principles, and concepts used in moral thinking.

Another version of the use of theory is to apply the four principles of Tom Beauchamp and Jim Childress's book (beneficence, non-maleficence, justice, and autonomy—the so-called Georgetown Mantra) to arrive at the correct answer.[11] In ethics rounds in hospitals, the poor resident or attending physician asked to comment on a case will invariably start by listing these four principles on the blackboard and will then mention aspects of the case touched by each of the principles. Then the discussion of what to do begins and continues for the next hour, with no mention whatsoever of the principles (much less any decision-procedure for balancing them to get the right answer).

To the view that knowledge of such principles or theories is important to being an ethical person, there is a standing challenge to all outside theorists by inside bioethicists: prove just one case, just one, where a person needs to know ethical theory to get the right answer and where virtually everyone in medicine or philosophy would agree (there would be that insight of, "Aha! Now I see what I didn't before!") that knowing the theory was the integral part in getting the previously unrevealed right answer. Many cases exist where people know the right answer and where ethicists use theories to redescribe the case in the appropriate theoretical terms, but this does not win the prize, being merely semantic redescription.[12]

Inside bioethicists come to this knowledge having sometimes been wounded by their training in graduate school, or perhaps better, their lack of training. Occasionally, some Ph.D. in philosophy or religion gets thrown right into a medical department or hospital and is asked immediately to help make a decision about DNR policy or testing for HIV infection. Almost certainly, the graduate program he recently attended has provided nothing that will help him make such decisions.

Outside bioethicists, of course, think inside ethicists are *only* interested in cases, never in critiquing a whole pattern of cases or of stepping back to see the big picture. Outside bioethicists see themselves as futurists, as theorists, as Socratic gadflies. Being such a gadfly is often a virtue for three special kinds of outside bioethicists, the political activist, the religious bioethicist, and the feminist bioethicist.

Although he is a rare bird in bioethics, often unpopular, and never an inside bioethicist, a political activist in bioethics constantly critiques physicians and the medical system. For example, he may rail against genetic discrimination in applying for jobs or medical insurance. He may complain about pharmaceutical companies giving medical students and residents free lunches and gifts (medical students get a free lunch from someone almost every day). He may complain about physicians accepting free trips financed by medical-supply companies to the Caribbean with fancy hotel rooms and well-stocked bars. He may complain about medical journals soliciting expensive ads from pharmaceutical companies and about doctors selling drugs and Amway products (Amway products!) from their offices. Such an outside ethicist is never asked to be on a hospital ethics committee.

Outside bioethicists who are publicly religious usually are conservative, for example, the Christian political conservative or the orthodox Jew. These ethicists are outside bioethicists because their primary allegiance is not to medicine but to God. As such, they may believe in certain absolute moral rules, for example, that abortions and physician-assisted killing are always wrong. Like other outside bioethicists, they are not primarily concerned with getting specific cases right or with building a professional consensus with other (mostly secular) bioethicists. What makes them allies with graduate philosophy professors is their common belief in more general, guiding moral principles or theoretical ideals.

Although the newest arrival in outside bioethics is the feminist, their numbers are growing. Emboldened by the popularity of the new "ethics of care" based on the work of Carol Gilligan and other feminist theoreticians in ethics, such bioethicists eschew the old emphasis on autonomy, rights, and cost-benefit analysis for a sensitivity to relationships, family affairs, and issues of gender. They may or may not be political, but if so, will bring a critique of patriarchy and sexism to their work (it is possible to combine all these kinds of "outside-nesses" as a bioethicist: politically active, religious, feminist).

Outside ethicists think inside ethicists too beholden to physicians or a hospital. They think that ethics consultants will agree with those who pay them for their consultations. It is unlikely that such a consultant will write anything too radical about the nature of medicine or be the first to blow the whistle on some practice in her home institution. Indeed, inside medical ethicists may be asked (or be assumed to be willing to give) "ethics cover" to the home institution when it is under attack, as in the Baby Fae case.[13]

Inside bioethicists are vulnerable to the charge of being an in-group and canaries all singing the same song. Inside bioethicists are very interested in certifying both themselves and newcomers as official bioethicists, with the implication that those who are uncertified are, well, . . . "uncertified."

Inside medical ethicists, when they publish, publish for each other. They have gone the way of philosophy and all the traditional fields: publishing only in specialty journals peer-reviewed by other (inside) bioethicists. Unfortunately, nobody much reads these articles, except inside bioethicists and their students. As Daniel Callahan has lamented, the early decades of bioethicists found bioethicists publishing in general, widely read publications, such as op-eds in national newspapers, but now that is rarely done.[14]

Inside bioethicists, especially when they are physicians, resent that so much of bioethics is represented by nonphysicians ("let's put the 'medical' back in 'medical ethics,'" they urge).[15] They think that medicine has its own internal moral values and admire the writings in this regard of Leon Kass and Edmund Pellegrino.[16] In so doing they soft-pedal the elitism contained in the way such writers extoll "ancient Greek values" (which, after all, were antidemocratic and accepted human slavery without criticism), while trying to maintain medicine on an ancient, noble tradition that is, frankly, built on a sense of noblesse oblige and whose obligations make little sense without it.

External bioethicists see things differently. Physician and bioethicist inside the University of Chicago and La Rabida Hospital John Lantos puts the conflict this way:

> Modern bioethics is dominated by nonphysicians. The conflict between an internal ethic of the profession and an external ethic for the profession energizes one of the more interesting debates in the field of bioethics. Simply stated, the question is whether medicine is primarily and intrinsically a moral enterprise, with its own internal values and norms, or whether it is primarily a technical and scientific enterprise that is morally neutral until society or culture or individual patients bring values that imbue it with moral purpose.[17]

(To return briefly to the topic of chapter 8, concerning the proper goals of medicine, it is interesting to note that both inside and outside bioethicists have argued that medical ethics can be set right when we discover such goals. But, again, I believe that the two will never agree on just what those goals are.)

It goes without saying that inside bioethicists abhor controversy in bioethics.[18] They are not of John Stuart Mill's persuasion that truth is best

forged in a spirited discussion of all possible points of view, no matter how outrageous some points of view may seem at first. Outside bioethicists, tending to
be academics not in hospital clinics, are more likely to be comfortable allowing
all sides of an issue to be heard.

The 1999 appointment of Australian bioethicist Peter Singer to Princeton
University's Center for Bioethics has become a bellwether for these two kinds
of bioethicists. Singer defends philosophically respectable views about animal
rights, aggressive treatment of severely impaired babies, and end-of-life medical treatment. Inside bioethicists generally distance themselves from Singer's
views, as animal rights is not popular inside medicine and few physicians will
publicly agree with Singer's views about impaired babies (although some will do
so privately). Outside bioethicists are far more likely to at least have their students read Singer, even if they end up criticizing his views.

The two kinds of bioethicist are mirrored in the opposing ways that a hospital ethics committee (HEC) functions. Perhaps more accurately, the real contrast is between two kinds of people who compose an HEC. People are often
appointed to an HEC because they have a particular point of view, for example, they are all sympathetic to the beliefs and mission of a Catholic hospital or
they are likely to defer to what a powerful physician says. Such committees
function like a well-oiled rubber-stamping machine. Rarely, an HEC may have
an outside ethicist, in which case, the committee might have trouble gaining
credibility inside the hospital. Under these circumstances, it is likely that no
cases will be referred to the committee. If HECs reflect the real pluralism in
bioethics, they will have an outside bioethicist (or a community member who
fulfills this "outsider" role). However, most are composed of inside bioethicists.

The two ways that HECs function here reflect the continuing problems that
have troubled them from their start. One such problem concerns their function: Is it to help physicians from the viewpoint of ordinary morality or to help
physicians fine-tune the internal morality of medicine?

A COMPROMISE?

The future of bioethics would be better if a new, synthetic breed of bioethicist
were to emerge, one with a foot in both camps. Bioethics cannot be based only
on cases, but it also cannot be based only on theory.

In truth, it is important to know some ethical theory in doing bioethics, even
in doing cases in hospitals and even if its importance is not what is implied in
graduate schools. For example, consider the rule of rescue, one of the most famous ideas that has originated in bioethics. This rule, which was named by the

bioethicist Albert Jonsen, refers to the strong social tendency to give an identified person rather than anonymous people a scarce medical resource. Equally needy and equally deserving, unidentified, "statistical" people don't get admitted to the system, appear on television, or get rescued.

Countless examples exist of the rule of rescue. When the plight of a small child trapped in a deep well is followed closely on television, thousands will contribute time and money for the rescue effort. Meanwhile, the stories of many other, equally deserving people in danger do not receive television coverage—and these people are not rescued and they die. So a cute, photogenic white girl gets on television to plead for a heart transplant—one girl among the fifty thousand who could use such a transplant each year.[19] Although UNOS (United Network for Organ Sharing) determines criteria of who will ultimately get such a transplant, to get listed one must have the money to pay for it, and the rule of rescue usually is invoked in such cases to raise the money.

With organ transplants, the rule of rescue has been used for nearly three decades to save a few children in organ failure. One infamous example occurred in 1982, when hospital administrator Charles Fiske blatantly manipulated the media at a press conference to obtain a liver donor for his daughter Jamie.

The criteria that drive the rule of rescue are usually irrelevant, trivial, or muddleheaded. Who gets to live shouldn't be decided by who gets on television and, hence, by who is most photogenic. Who gets to live shouldn't be decided by who has been admitted to a hospital, who has gotten into the system, or who has a father with access to reporters.

Furthermore, the rule of rescue can mean that unaccustomed people make decisions about who lives and who dies. As newspaper and television editors quickly found out, the rule of rescue may replace the "God committee" with the newsroom editor. Finally, the greatest problem with the rule of rescue is that for every identified person who is saved, there are countless anonymous patients who are not.

Most of these problems are well known in bioethics, but what is less appreciated is the fact that the rule of rescue represents a clash between two kinds of ethical theories: the ethics of care, focusing on relations with identified people, and impartialist theories, such as Kantian ethics or utilitarianism, that entail treating everyone the same, identified or not.

This kind of theoretical clash is not unique to the rule of rescue or its many examples. Many cases in medical ethics are brought to their sharpest tension by emphasizing the clash between two large theoretical points of view. Consider another example of such a class of ethical theories: a pulmonary resident discovers that he missed a small lesion three months previously on the X ray of a forty-eight-year-old patient. The patient now has level 4, untreatable cancer.

The patient says, "I guess that cancer just grew out of nowhere because it wasn't there three months ago." Should the resident tell the patient the truth?

Consequentialists often argue that he should not because little good will occur to the patient at this time. For deontologists such as Kant, however, the answer is clear: the patient must be told the truth. Why? The only universalizable rule is, "Always tell patients the truth." Such a rule is the basis of trust and of treating patients as "ends in themselves." If the physician were the patient, he also would want to know the truth. The resident may *feel* that he shouldn't reveal the truth, but his reason will tell him what his duty is.

As said, such clashes between Kantian ethics (deontology) and utilitarianism (consequentialism), or between both and other theories, are quite common. Having thought about them before one enters medicine, and even while one does medicine, is obviously a good thing for students and physicians, and even more obviously, *necessary* training for bioethicists.

BIOETHICAL FERRYMEN

In Indian religion, noble ferrymen help enlightened souls cross over a river to Nirvana. Sometimes called a *bodishattva*, this being is half human, half divine. Although he could cross over forever, he lingers on the river, not becoming fully divine, to help other humans complete their journey.

Although help from *bodishattvas* is not likely in re-creating bioethics, it is possible that some merely human people can bridge the two worlds, shuttling back and forth. Yet this "ferrying" task may call for superhuman qualities, since a bioethicist with a foot in both camps may not be fully loved in either. Such a "bioethical ferryman" will be regarded as too inside for the outside department and too outside for the inside department.

Such ferrymen could reinvigorate bioethics because real thinking occurs best when motivated by real cases. Resolution of such cases, in turn, is always helped by knowledge of what has been done in the past, the ethical reasoning behind such past actions, and what others do in similar cases around the world (and again, *why* they do so). It is even possible that such a "re-created bioethics" will birth a new ethical theory.

Creating this new breed of bioethics will take a new kind of Bioethics Ph.D. program. Philosophy and theology graduate programs are hopelessly oriented toward protecting disciplinary boundaries and as such, are antithetical and hostile to real *inter*disciplinary work[20] (one could also say that about medical sociology, literature and medicine, history of medicine, medical economics, and medical anthropology).

My hope is that a true, interdisciplinary Ph.D. program is created. There are already a number of excellent master's programs, but they rarely have assistantships and fellowships. Such a Ph.D. program would need to offer assistantships and tuition scholarships, because otherwise good students cannot afford to study bioethics over four years. That means that graduate students would have to assist/teach undergraduate courses in bioethics, which means that such courses would be in the bioethics and not in the philosophy or religion departments. This, of course, would result in a battle, because the departments currently getting the tuition and assistantships from undergraduate courses would fight to keep them. So the politics of setting up an interdisciplinary Ph.D. program in bioethics are considerable.

Nevertheless, it could be a wonderful program. My fantasy is that there would be graduate courses in history of medicine, medicine and literature (students would read Abraham Verghese's *My Own Country* and Richard Selzer's *Letters to a Young Surgeon*), ethical theory, medical economics, medical sociology, public health and ethics, evidence-based medical reasoning, in addition to a core course in the history of bioethics and a half-dozen specialized courses on particular topics such as genetic testing, assisted reproduction, and death and dying. All this would be intertwined with clinical conferences in hospitals that discuss ethical issues in real cases. Such conferences would start the very first year. There would be a mandatory, one-year internship in a hospital, around which a doctoral dissertation would be sandwiched.

As I said, a fantasy.

NOTES

1. My involvement in bioethics began with a letter in the *Hastings Center Report* 2, no. 4 (September 1972), 6.

2. At UAB, medical ethics is a required, letter-graded course of thirty-two to forty hours for the 165 first-year medical students each year. I've taught this course since 1977.

3. Trisha Macnair, "Career Focus: Medical Ethics," *British Medical Journal* 319, no. S2 (2 October 1999): 7212–4. *BMJ* is on the web in its entirety at www.bmj.com.

4. Albert Jonsen, "Why Has Bioethics Become Boring?" Lifetime Achievement Award talk, American Society for Bioethics and Humanities, 30 October 1999, Philadelphia, Pennsylvania.

5. Nancy M. King, "Who Ate the Apple? A Commentary on the Core Competencies Report," *HEC Forum* 11, no. 2 (June 1999): 174.

6. People may think of medical centers and hospitals as the same, but they are not. A medical center encompasses many schools, such as medicine, nursing, public health, and dentistry, and probably several hospitals. In the schools, students take courses in

1 9 6   RE-CREATING MEDICINE

large lecture rooms for the first two years and have little contact with patients. So one can easily be a bioethicist teaching in such classrooms and not be in a hospital. Most bioethicists encounter students only in a classroom, not in a hospital.

7. Carl Elliot, *A Philosophical Disease: Bioethics, Culture, and Identity* (New York: Routledge, 1999), xxii.

8. Macnair, "Career Focus: Medical Ethics," www.bmj.com.

9. Within the past year, nearly 40 percent of physicians reported that they sometimes deceive insurance companies to help patients obtain coverage for needed services. See the abstract presented by the AMA's Institute for Ethics at the Association for Health Services Research Annual Meeting, June 1999, *Journal of the American Medical Association* (30 August 1999).

10. Stephen Toulmin, "The Tyranny of Principles," *Hastings Center Report* 11, no. 6 (December 1981): 31–9. See also his justly famous, "How Medicine Saved the Life of Ethics," *Perspectives in Biology and Medicine* 25 (1982): 736–50.

11. Tom Beauchamp and Jim Childress, *The Principles of Medical Ethics*, fourth edition (Englewood Cliffs, N.J.: Prentice-Hall, 1998). Both authors have a connection to Georgetown University, hence the name.

12. There is also a more brutal challenge by hospital-based physicians: come over to our hospital and round with us one day, and we'll describe the ethical issues of the cases that day. Then we'll see how your theories and principles help us solve our cases. Few, if any, theorists ever accept such a challenge: most like to stay in their offices and write about ethics.

13. See Gregory E. Pence, "Baby Fae and Baby Theresa," *Classic Cases in Medical Ethics: Accounts of the Cases that Shaped Medical Ethics*, third edition (New York: Mc-Graw-Hill, 2000), chapter 13.

14. Daniel Callahan, "The Hastings Center and the Early Years of Bioethics," *Kennedy Institute of Ethics Journal* 9, no. 1 (March 1999): 69.

15. John Lantos, *Do We Still Need Doctors?* (New York: Routledge, 1997), 161.

16. Leon Kass, *Towards a More Natural Science* (New York: Viking, 1987); Edmund Pellegrino, "Ethics," *Journal of the American Medical Association* 275 (1996): 1807–9.

17. Lantos, *Do We Still Need Doctors?*, 161.

18. One recent meltdown in bioethics occurred after one bioethicist on *60 Minutes* accused many others at other institutions of retrieving organs from patients who were legally still persons and not dead. The controversy surrounded implementation of the so-called Pittsburgh protocol to use non-heart-beating cadaver donors for organ harvest at the Cleveland Clinic and at the University of Wisconsin Medical Center. See Robert Arnold and Stuart Younger, "Back to the Future: Obtaining Organs from Non-Heart-Beating Cadavers," *Kennedy Institute of Ethics* 3, no. 2 (June 1993): 106, and the Institute of Medicine, *Non-Heart-Beating Organ Transplantation: Medical and Ethical Issues in Procurement* (Washington, D.C.: National Academy Press, 1997), 23–5.

19. Cynthia Fox, "Heartless," *Life* (November 1999): 124.

20. The antipathy of graduate programs in philosophy and theology to case-oriented bioethics is well known. Popular courses in bioethics, which bring in the tuition dollars that pay the expensive salaries of the graduate professors, are relegated to graduate students who've never had a course in bioethics. This is how the world turns.

10

CONCLUSIONS AND REFLECTIONS

His achievements are written in imperishable letters in the annals of modern surgical practice, and there are thousands now living, and succeeding thousands in generations of women unborn, who will have reason to rise up and call him blessed. Originally a country practitioner in Alabama, he succeeded by sheer force of unaided genius, and by the characteristics of thoroughness, simplicity, and ingenuity of character and methods in introducing such improvements in the surgery of some of the most obscure and previously irremediable diseases of women, as to have brought about something like a revolution in the methods and results of practice. . . . The greatest success which any surgeon of genius can hope to achieve is to be able to definitely and largely add to the power of surgery to save life, to relieve misery, and to effect cure. This success Marion Sims attained is a degree which few can hope to attain. He was known in all the capitals in Europe and in all he has left an enduring monument and bequeathed a legacy for which suffering humanity will ever feel cause to feel grateful.

—Obituary of J. Marion Sims, *British Medical Journal*, 1884,
   quoted in Seale Harris, *Woman's Surgeon: The Life Story of J. Marion Sims*

Can we learn from the past? Every time I enter the Reynolds Library for the History of Medicine at UAB, I pass a stained glass window purchased by J. Marion Sims and his family for their favorite church in New York City—after he had established the first women's hospital there and become world famous. On Fifth Avenue in the Upper East Side of Manhattan, a statue of Sims greets people in front of the New York Academy of Medicine. At UAB, in the Center for Advanced Medical Study, there is a painting of him operating and there is (appropriately) the J. Marion Sims endowed chair in Obstetrics and Gynecology. Despite these reminders, few people in New York or Alabama know the real story of Sims, how he fought to change the status quo of medicine of his time, or what he endured. Few women today would think of Sims as a hero who helped them.

Sims was not a perfect physician and is a tarnished hero because he did not rise above the racism in Alabama of the 1860s. But he should also not be ignored, not only because of his pioneering focus on the special medical problems of women but also because of his pioneering efforts to overcome infertility. We should realize that these bold efforts were met in his time with moral ridicule.

Likewise, the successes of reproductive medicine today seem lost amidst the growing chorus of cries for regulation. While allowing financial incentives to continue unregulated seems inconceivable to many in bioethics and medicine, such incentives have nevertheless been the fuel that has brought us those fifty thousand new American babies. Just as women all over the world traveled long distances to be Sims's patients, so infertile couples from all over the world come to the United States for a chance at having a child of their own.

Concerning organ donation, our heads are still ostrich-like, under the sand. We persist in believing that more education will awaken a huge pool of dormant altruism in people, even as modern life gets more stressful and demanding. The number of needless deaths, coupled with the number of organs needlessly lost, makes rewarded organ transfers reasonable to consider now, especially from cadaveric donors. And it is not as if our present system is pure and snow white. How many decades will need to pass before we can say that our present policy has failed all those who have died waiting?

The past century and recent decades have shown that people get nervous about expanding parental choices about having children. Such nervousness is predictable, but let's make policy on what we know of people in our neighborhood and at work, not on what we see on TV shows or find in fiction.

The idea of really being able to choose whether and when to have a child is very new in human consciousness. We forget how new birth control really is and how cumbersome it is to use. The Alan Guttmacher Institute, the most reputable source for data on pregnancy and birth control, estimates that two-thirds of U.S. women will be unintentionally pregnant at some time in their lives.[1] This is hardly a statistic from a country where births are routinely planned and chosen.

Parental choice about kinds of children also scares people. It is therefore no surprise that the idea of choosing specific traits for children is also met with such resistance and skepticism, especially by those who believe that magic happens when the genetic spindle turns and when chromosomes mix to form the genotype of a human embryo.

In reality, things are much more dismal than I described in chapter 5 in the upbeat "Dear Kids" letter from (and to) the future. We have not had one true success with individualized genetic therapy. There seems to be a problem with the platform that introduces the genetic change. Viruses are too unstable, and the hope now is for an artificial chromosome that will add on to existing ones and carry genetic corrections.[2]

I attended the national meetings of the American Genetics Society in Denver in the fall of 1998. Graduate students had hundreds of poster sessions with color photographs of children born with congenital diseases caused by hundreds of known genetic diseases. I was shocked to see how much misery is caused by random genetic causation.

My sense is that, if you saw the pictures like me of all these children and all the terrible things genetic diseases do, you would also agree that we are being too timid in seeking cures for these conditions. We fear vague, abstract things while every day terrible genetic diseases slam down kids and families. Like the historical lesson about AID, the lesson here is that being cautious about dangers must be balanced against the lives of those who die each year from genetic disease.

Perhaps we need more than the "Speaker for the Future" (mentioned in chapter 5). Perhaps we need a "Speaker for the Genetically Afflicted" (to speed up genetic therapies), a "Speaker for Those-Waiting-for-Transplants" (to advocate compensated cadaveric donation), and a "Speaker for Unrescued Patients" (to promote impartial access for all to medical care).

The most important issue left unresolved in this book is one that grows more urgent every day in the newest branches of medicine: How much risk should physicians permit competent adults to take? Indeed, it also ran through many of the book's chapters, from competent adults selling kidneys or parts of livers to young women selling eggs, from patients who want to take risks with drugs to enhance athletic performance to patients who will one day want to take risks with genetic enhancements.

I do not believe that the traditional, paternalistic role of physicians is suited to being the gatekeeper of approved theories of the good life. Lawrence Schneiderman and Nancy Jecker, Leon Kass and Daniel Callahan, as well as Edmund Pellegrino[3] would have us turn to the past for the ancient role of the wise physician who can make such judgments, but I suspect that role is more mythical than factual. In terms of chapter 9, are the approved views of the good life to be determined by the conservative, internal morality of medicine or by the outside society upon medicine? Are the proper kinds of risk taking to be determined by the internal excellences and practices of medicine or by the risk takers in our general society? If the former, how does that square with the ideal of shared decision making between patient and physician as moral equals?

Obviously, we need a consistent philosophical theory of which risks are acceptable in medicine for competent adults to take. I stress "consistent" because we now allow such adults to take grave risks in trying to beat cancer and we allow them to donate a kidney to an unrelated stranger. Given that, what kinds of risk are allowed for motives that are financially self-interested but that have beneficial consequences to others (selling organs, eggs, sperm)? Is this kind of risk different than when such self-interested actions have no beneficial consequences to others (genetic self-enhancement)? Finally, if adults are making children take such risks (cloning, germ-line therapy, and enhancement), how much risk is then acceptable and why? If we cannot agree on answers of content to these questions, can we agree on a process, that is, on which professional or committee should decide? These are the questions that a consistent theory of risk must answer.

As the year 2000 begins, we are on the edge of exciting new frontiers in medicine. As I have argued in this book, I hope that we will not be too timid in reevaluating the traditional moral rules of medicine. If we are not, it will be easier to get there.

NOTES

1. Alan Guttmacher Institute, *Teenage Sexual and Reproductive Behavior: Facts in Brief* (New York: Alan Guttmacher Institute, 1993).

2. "The Last Taboo" (editorial) and "How to Make an Artificial Chromosome," *New Scientist* 2209 (23 October 1999): 3–4.

3. Edmund Pellegrino, "Ethics," *Journal of the American Medical Association* 275 (1996): 1807–9.

INDEX

ABOUT THE AUTHOR

Gregory E. Pence has been a faculty member of the University of Alabama at Burmingham (UAB) since January 1976. In addition to teaching in the Department of Philosophy, he teaches a course in medical ethics to all first-year students in UAB's School of Medicine. Professor Pence graduated cum laude in Philosophy in 1970 from the College of William and Mary in Williamsburg, Virginia, and earned his Ph.D. in 1974 from New York University in New York City.

Dr. Pence's writings include *Classic Cases in Medical Ethics: Accounts of the Cases that Shaped Medical Ethics* (McGraw-Hill, 3rd edition 2000), *Who's Afraid of Human Cloning?* (Rowman & Littlefield, 1997), and, with G. Lynn Stevens, *Seven Dilemmas in World Religions* (Paragon House, 1994). He has edited *Classic Works in Medical Ethics: Core Philosophical Readings* (McGraw-Hill, 1997) and *Flesh of My Flesh: The Ethics of Cloning Humans* (Rowman & Littlefield, 1998). In 1994 he received UAB's most prestigious teaching award, the Ingalls Award for Best Teaching in the Classroom. He is also director of the Early Medical School Acceptance Program (EMSAP) at UAB, a BS/MD program.